LOSE ⸻

Copyri⸻

The right of Eddie Bojtler to ⸻
been asserted by him ⸻ ⸻ ⸻ight,
Designs a⸻ ⸻ 1988.

All rights reserved. No part of this publication may be reproduced, stored in a retrieval system, or transmitted in any form or by any means, electronic, mechanical, photocopying, recording or otherwise, without the prior written permission of the copyright owner.

ISBN: 978-0-9558105-0-3

Design by David Jenner of Esquire Print Ltd.
Diamond Works, Maidstone Road, Nettlestead, Maidstone, Kent ME18 5HP

Printed and bound in Great Britain by Trade Print Europe Limited

Published by IntaShape Ltd
Diamond Works, Maidstone Road, Nettlestead, Maidstone, Kent ME18 5HP

NUTRITION: The nutritional values are approximations and can be affected by the unknown composition of some manufactured foods and uncertainty in the dietary database.

IMPORTANT: The IntaShape inch loss plan is based on the average results of thousands of men and women and you could lose more or less inches than those shown. Anybody with specific dietary needs, or the elderly, pregnant women, young children and those suffering from immune deficiency disease should consult their GP before changing their diets.

REAL PEOPLE... REAL RESULTS

The testimonials shown below are all of real people who have got results with the IntaShape Plan. Their photos and results are real and all have signed testimonials to this effect.

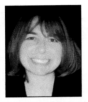

DONNA ROW
Administrator

Lost 10 inches, 9 pounds and 3.4% fat mass in 6 weeks.

"The great thing about IntaShape is it involves so much common sense."

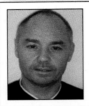

STEVE MYERS
IT Manager

Lost 7 inches, 9 pounds and 2.6% fat mass in just 5 weeks.

"Simple and straight forward."

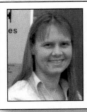

SAM BESSANT
Learning & Development Group Leader

Lost 9 inches, 7.5 pounds and 2.3% fat mass in just 5 weeks.

"IntaShape has lead me to a much healthier lifestyle."

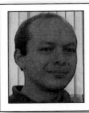

JULIAN BRYANT
IT Business Analyst

Lost 9 inches, 6 pounds and 2% fat mass in 6 weeks.

"Realistic & easy to follow."

REAL PEOPLE... REAL RESULTS

The testimonials shown below are all of real people who have got results with the IntaShape Plan. Their photos and results are real and all have signed testimonials to this effect.

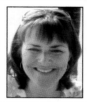

DEBBIE JONES
Company Secretary

Lost 7.5 inches, 7 pounds and 2% fat mass in 6 weeks.

"This is a no-nonsense, sensible plan that becomes a way of life"

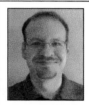

DAVID LEWIS
Web Developer

Lost 6 inches, 6.5 pounds and 2.6% fat mass in just 5 weeks.

"Simplicity itself: you will see results."

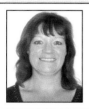

JAYNE LUCKENS
Export Packer

Lost 7 inches, 7 pounds and 3.1% fat mass in just 5 weeks.

"I now have my social life back and still can lose inches"

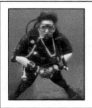

LAURA EDWARDS
Office Supervisor & Scuba Diver

Lost 9 inches, 10 pounds and 3.9% fat mass in 6 weeks.

"I never thought that by the first 6 weeks I would have lost so much size!"

REAL PEOPLE... REAL RESULTS

The testimonials shown below are all of real people who have got results with the IntaShape Plan. Their photos and results are real and all have signed testimonials to this effect.

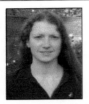

RUTH COOPER
Microbiologist
Lost 8 inches, 8 pounds and 2.9% fat mass in 6 weeks.

"Easy to follow and really helped me to focus"

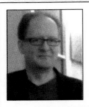

GRAHAME DANBY
Scientist
Lost 5.5 inches, 8 pounds and 2.7% fat mass in just 5 weeks.

"IntaShape is based on good sense and realism"

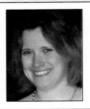

CHRISTINE JOHNSON
Civil Servant
Lost 6 inches, 10 pounds and 2.9% fat mass in 6 weeks.

"A complete lifestyle change. I would recommend this programme to anyone"

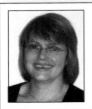

DAWN CURRAN
HR Manager
Lost 6 inches, 5 pounds and 2.5% fat mass in just 5 weeks.

"Realistic, allowing for special occasions and very motivational"

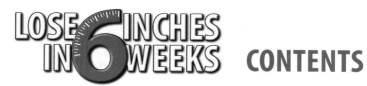 **CONTENTS**

ABOUT THE AUTHOR

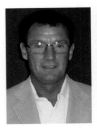

Eddie Bojtler is the author of this book and the creator of the IntaShape inch loss plan. This book is the result of 10 years of hands on experience in the field of weight management.

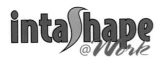

Eddie's background includes working for two Global Pharmaceutical companies to take their workforce through the IntaShape at Work programme.

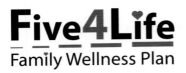

His Five4Life Family Wellness Plan was used to help 500 families in the North West of England improve their lifestyle through the government funded Sure Start.

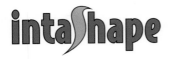

He has trained hundreds of health & fitness professionals to deliver the IntaShape plan to thousands of gym members within the fitness industry.

Eddie actually started in fitness spending more than 15 years in the elite Army Physical Training Corps were he reached the rank of warrant officer class one. He has been the British Bobsleigh Trainer. Eddie has also trained athletes to international level and appeared on 'This is Your Life' as the trainer to the World Water Skiing Champion Liz Hobbs.

His first venture into the world of weight management came in 1989 when he took up the position of Health & Fitness Manager for a new and large gym complex where the goal of most gym members was to lose weight. Five years later he set up his own personal lifestyle coaching company with nearly six hundred personal clients, most of whom wanted to lose weight. It was here that the blueprint to the IntaShape inch loss plan started.

FOOD FOR THOUGHT

Several years ago my brother changed jobs and with the new job came a brand new diesel car. The first time he had to drive his brand new diesel car to a garage to fill up with fuel, guess what? He filled his brand new diesel car up with petrol!

As soon as others in the company had realised what he had done he received some very interesting text messages. One was from his boss that asked him this... *"How could you put the wrong type of fuel into your car?"* A very good question!

Here's an even better one...how could anyone put the wrong type of food into their body, especially if they want to become slimmer?

Today we are constantly bombarded with different messages on how to eat healthily and what we need to do to lose weight. Unfortunately, these messages can often lead to a state of personal confusion, especially when one piece of advice is the direct opposite of another. Shown next are several popular suggestions about what you need to do to become slimmer:

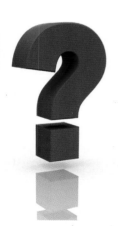

- Don't eat after eight o'clock at night.
- Don't snack between meals.
- Don't mix carbohydrate with protein.
- Cut out bread and potatoes.
- Alcohol contains no fat.
- Eat more healthy fats.
- Sugar is bad for you.
- If you're not sweating you're not exercising hard enough.
- Go for the burn.

You are about to uncover how much truth there is behind these statements. In the process you will discover what you have to do to lose 6 inches of fat in 6 weeks and how to keep these inches off afterwards.

Eddie Bojtler

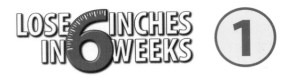

THE WEIGHT LOSS TRAP

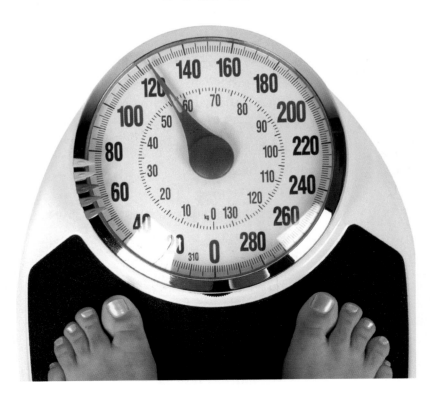

JUST LOSE WEIGHT

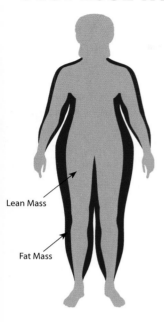

Lean Mass

Fat Mass

The general advice for those who are overweight is to lose weight. It does not matter how you lose the weight; as long as you lose weight. If you're losing two pounds a week in weight then you must be doing the right thing.

Of course it matters how you lose weight. If you lose weight from the wrong places it will make all the difference to the way you look, feel and whether the pounds will go back on again with interest. And this is where you need to be aware of the difference between a bad change in body composition and a good change in body composition. In other words you can lose weight with unhealthy consequences or you can lose weight healthily.

BAD CHANGE IN BODY COMPOSITION

Look at your body in a different light. On the inside is that slim, trim person trying to break free. This is called lean mass and your lean mass includes water, muscle and energy stored within your muscles. Water, muscle & muscle energy are essential for your body to function efficiently.

Completely covering your lean mass is a dense coat called fat mass. Fat mass is made up of billions of tiny fat cells, collectively holding thousands of fat calories.

Carrying too much fat mass spoils your shape; hides lean mass, makes your body flabby and can lead to health problems such as high blood pressure and an increased risk of coronary heart disease.

A bad change in body composition takes place
when you lose lean mass that you have on the inside,
without losing much fat mass on the outside.

In simple terms you lose the healthy area of your body whilst holding on to the unhealthy area.

YOU LOSE WEIGHT EVERY DAY

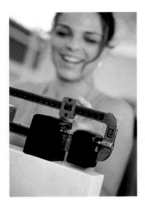

Each day you lose weight. Most of this weight is lost from water and energy from inside your lean mass. Only a few ounces are lost from your fat mass.

Up to two thirds of your body is water. For every pint of water you drink, you gain one pound in weight. Alternatively, for every pint of water you lose, you lose one pound in weight. The main indicator of a bad change in body composition is rapid weight loss in the first few days (up to five pounds), with no significant increase in activity levels.

A continued reduction in lean mass leads to saggy skin (*"you've lost too much weight"* is the cry.) In reality, it is the loss of lean mass that creates this and not the loss of fat mass. So now you have to start doing toning up exercises to replace the lean mass you lost through the bad weight loss.

A reduction in lean mass can lead to an increase in cellulite. Cellulite is not helped when lean mass is reduced and fat mass is increased. This can lead to poorer circulation in specific areas like the thighs. Replacing your lean mass while decreasing your fat mass can help you win the battle against cellulite.

Furthermore, a reduction in lean mass levels reduces the total number of calories your body uses as energy each day therefore you should consume fewer calories. You can also lose strength, vitality and your metabolic rate lowers, which makes it more difficult to lose weight later.

BRITISH HEART FOUNDATION'S MAGAZINE

So you want to lose weight... for good!
"Secondly, losing weight quickly involves losing essential water and muscle as well as fat. So, although the scales may read less, your body has not lost much fat! Thirdly, your metabolic rate slows down and it becomes even harder to lose weight. Gradual weight loss is really the safest and most effective way"

You now reach a point when you find it very difficult to continue to keep making progress. It's as though your body has reached a set point and you cannot lose any more weight.

Eventually, when you do decide to stop following the diet and go back to your old eating habits, you consume more calories. This allows your lean mass levels to be restored and your weight should return to your starting weight. However, if you have not been controlling your total fat intake during the diet, your fat mass will have increased and you will have gained additional weight from fat.

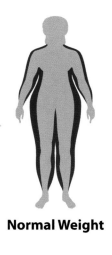

Normal Weight

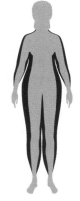

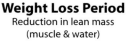

Weight Loss Period
Reduction in lean mass
(muscle & water)

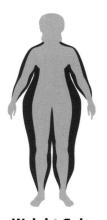

Weight Gain
Restored lean mass
(muscle & water)
plus increase in fat mass.

Unhealthy weight loss is caused through diets or poor eating habits that contain insufficient calories for good health. These diets or food plans are often low in carbohydrate and sometimes protein. To prevent a loss of lean mass you should consume the correct amount of both carbohydrate and protein. It does not make any sense to consume more calories than your body needs, as this will only exacerbate fat gain.

Of course you will lose more weight on a lower calorie diet like the cabbage soup diet. Unfortunately, this additional weight loss will be the result of a reduction in your lean mass and not just from your fat mass. The next couple of pages provide two disturbing examples of the emotional effect caused through bad weight loss.

IT'S YOUR FAULT!

In 1997 I went to visit a gym owner in Kent who was interested in taking on the IntaShape plan, or at least that's what I thought.

I arrived at the gym in good time and went up into reception, where I was met by a smiling receptionist. She said that Pete (the gym owner) was expecting me and could I take a seat for a few minutes.

Pete arrived, introduced himself and asked me into his office to discuss my programme. As I sat down the smiling receptionist also came into the office and sat down. Before I could say anything this lady exploded into life blaming me and people like me for ruining her life. Pete sat back and just watched.

The now angry receptionist went on to say that she had followed diets most of her life and all she had left was a load of saggy skin hanging down. She had contacted a number of the organisations whose diet she had followed, to ask how this had happened, but none had replied to her. As I was partly to blame for this could I explain to her why this had happened!

I asked her why she thought it was saggy skin that was hanging down. She said what else could it be and took off her tracksuit bottoms to show me her legs. The first thing that struck me was that her legs were totally out of proportion to the way she looked. Her legs were bigger than I expected to see and seemed to be covered in fat. I then asked if I could measure her fat mass using the fat mass callipers I had with me. She agreed for this to be done.

It is worth pointing out that by now I had experience of measuring fat mass, using the callipers, with hundreds of men and women. I measured her fat mass percentage as nearly 37 percent. This was five percent more than what a woman of her age should have to be graded as normal fat mass percentage. Yet, she claimed to have lost nearly eight stone in weight!

Although she must have lost some fat mass, it was obvious from looking at her body that she had also lost a massive amount of lean body tissue in the process and serious damage to her self-esteem. Fad diets offer you fast and effortless weight loss in the early days but there can be a very heavy price to pay later.

HOW COULD I HAVE BEEN SO STUPID!

A few years later I was in the middle of training six fitness professionals in a different gym to deliver the IntaShape programme to their members. We got to the part of the course that deals with measuring fat mass using the fat mass callipers. I asked for a volunteer so that I could measure their fat mass. Not all fitness professionals have experience using fat mass callipers and need to be shown.

One of the female members of the gym team said that she would like me to measure her fat mass. This came as a bit of a surprise, as she was the one having difficulty coming to terms with certain parts of the plan. I measured her fat mass using the callipers and this came out as normal for her age group and gender… no problem there, or so I thought.

When she realised what the outcome of her fat mass was she burst into tears in front of the whole group and said "how could I have been so stupid!"

This young lady has just graduated in Sports Science from university. She had kept her fat mass results taken at the university the year before, which she now showed to the whole group. Those measurements, taken one year earlier, were almost identical to the ones that I had just taken… so why was she so upset?

Since leaving university she had lost two stone in weight following a very popular low carbohydrate diet at the time, yet her fat mass had remained unchanged! She had lost weight from lean mass and not from fat mass.

She went on to say "I knew what was happening, it was clear that I was not losing fat mass, but I was so desperate to lose weight that I just kept on going!"

If you can actually learn to live without regularly using the scales, you will find that life is much easier. This is especially true for children who are now getting hooked at a young age on having to rely on the scales. It will only set them up for years of misery later.

It is a far healthier attitude to eat sensibly and be a bit more active and accept that there will be days when your weight will fluctuate. Go by the way your clothes fit and how you look in the mirror.

It's not the amount of weight you lose on any diet or weight loss programme that is the issue. It's the amount of fat you have lost that makes all the difference to the way you look and feel.

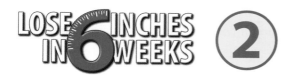

HOW TO
TARGET FAT

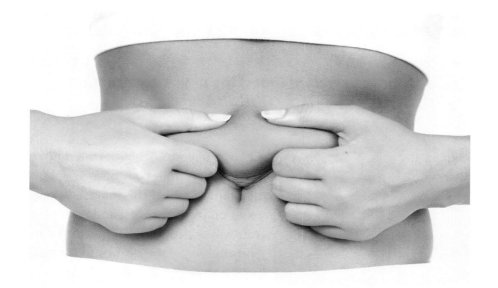

INCHES OR WEIGHT?

Today's current belief is that by losing a certain amount of weight, you will be losing the same proportion in inches. Thus, a five pound drop in weight is seen to be better than a three pound drop. The key is not the amount of weight you lose but the number of inches you lose in fat with that weight. Would you prefer to lose five pounds and three inches in fat, or lose five pounds and six inches in fat?

If you think about it, to drop a dress or trouser size you must lose x amount of inches or centimetres. Rather than looking to lose more weight quickly, look to lose more inches in fat. The quicker you shed inches or centimetres in flab, the faster you will fit comfortably into your new dress or trousers and the better you will look.

Nobody puts on their best beach outfit or jeans and runs up and down the beach or high street carrying a set of scales overhead shouting "look I am only nine stone!" Its how you look in your swimsuit or jeans that catches the eye.

It's not your weight that is the physical attraction,
IT'S YOUR SHAPE!

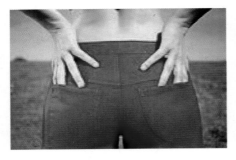

Changing your goal to shedding more inches in fat from your body will require a different mindset. This mindset is one that relies on the mirror first and not the scales. You will notice the changes in the mirror and the way your clothes fit, sometimes before they register on the scales.

How many mornings do you step onto the scales and do not like what you see? So you move the scales until you find a kinder spot! Now the only thing that has changed is the number on the scales. Your body is exactly the same as it was when you stepped on the scales in the first place.

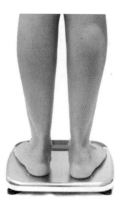

You must first be able to see the changes in the mirror before you step on the scales. This is the best way to know that you are losing inches from your fat mass. Better still; adopt the habit of using the mirror and the way your clothes fit, rather than just relying on the scales.

CREATE A GOOD CHANGE IN BODY COMPOSITION

A good change in body composition means that you become slimmer on the outside through a reduction in your fat mass, while holding onto your lean mass on the inside.

Now it could be that you don't need to lose any weight; you just want to shed a few unwanted inches and these principles will work just as well for you. Importantly you will be losing fat from your fat mass, while retaining essential water, muscle and muscle energy.

GUIDELINES FOR FAT INTAKE

Shown next are the daily guidelines for the amount of fat you should consume as an average each day. An average means that on some days you may have a lower fat intake, while other days you could have higher fat intake but the average over time would be as follows:

DAILY GUIDELINES FOR FAT FOR MEN & WOMEN

	Men	Women
Total fat	95 grams per day	70 grams
Total amount of saturated fat	30 grams per day	20 grams

ARE YOU LUCKY?

If you can lose more than 70 grams of fat each day as a woman, or 95 grams of fat each day as a man, without leading an active lifestyle, or exercise, then you have a good metabolic rate, and you are lucky in that respect.

To reduce your fat mass you need to consume fewer than 95 grams of fat a day as a man and 70 grams of fat a day as a woman. Simply by cutting your total fat intake to between 30-40 grams of fat per day you will achieve this.

The average man is expected to use 95 grams of fat per day as energy. This is 25 grams more than the average women and is one of the reasons why it is easier for the average man to lose more inches and weight than the average women.

LOSE INCHES BY NOT GOING HUNGRY

Hunger is your enemy, as you are more likely to eat too much when you feel very hungry. By consuming three low-fat, high-fibre meals a day, which, although are low in fat, actually make you feel full. In addition, two fresh fruit snacks a day between meals stop you from snacking on high-sugar/high-fat snacks.

Another advantage that you gain from consuming fresh fruit between meals is that your energy levels do not dip mid morning or mid afternoon. You also have the option of an additional evening snack, especially if you have had a physically active day.

Even though you will be consuming three meals a day, plus two to three snacks a day, your total fat intake will be fewer than 40 grams a day!

Regular physical activity is just as important as healthy eating and the two go hand in hand with this plan. The sections on Get Active and Fat Busting Activities will explain how you can easily combine everyday activities with the plan for food and drinks to target fat and lose 6 inches in 6 weeks.

TARGETING FAT

DAILY GUIDELINES FOR FAT INTAKE FOR WOMEN & MEN

	Women	*Men*
Total fat	*70 grams*	*95 grams*

**TO TARGET FAT LOSS YOU NEED TO KEEP YOUR
DAILY FAT INTAKE TO BETWEEN 30-40 GRAMS PER DAY.**

FAT LOST EACH DAY

WOMEN WILL LOSE BETWEEN 30-40 GRAMS OF FAT A DAY.

MEN WILL LOSE BETWEEN 55-65 GRAMS OF FAT A DAY.

**REGULAR PHYSICAL ACTIVITY WILL INCREASE
THE AMOUNT OF FAT YOU LOSE.**

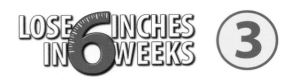

THE PLAN FOR
FOOD & DRINKS

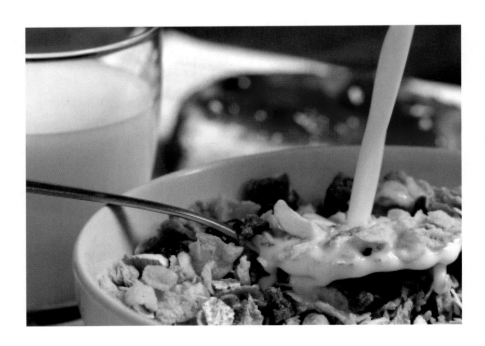

THE PLAN FOR FOOD & DRINKS

| Low Fat Breakfast | Morning Snack | Low Fat Lunch | Afternoon Snack | Low Fat Evening Meal | Evening Snack (Optional) | 2-3 Units |

THE PLAN FOR FOOD & DRINKS

1. **THREE LOW-FAT, HIGH-FIBRE, BALANCED MEALS PER DAY.**
    (A low-fat meal is any breakfast, lunch or evening meal with up to 10 grams of fat.)

    ---

2. **A MID-MORNING FRESH FRUIT SNACK.**

3. **A MID-AFTERNOON FRESH FRUIT SNACK.**

4. **AN EVENING SNACK IF YOU STILL FEEL HUNGRY.**

    ---

5. **CONSUMING NO MORE THAN TWO UNITS OF ALCOHOL PER DAY FOR WOMEN.**

6. **CONSUMING NO MORE THAN THREE UNITS OF ALCOHOL PER DAY FOR MEN.**

Total fat intake eating three meals and two to three snacks
is only between 30-40 grams of fat a day.

KEEPING YOU FOCUSSED AND MOTIVATED

Can you remember what you ate and drank two weeks ago? You need a simple tool to help you with this. Some programmes involving food use the food diary system. This is where you write down each day what you ate and drank.

Yet there is another way for you to keep control of what you eat and drink over the next 6 weeks. It's quick to complete, easy to use and actually helps you to make the best choices each day. Let's say that on day 1 of the programme you followed the plan for food and drinks to the letter.

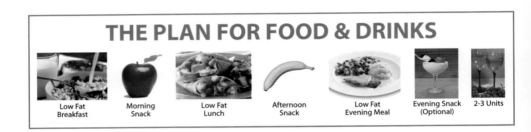

THE PLAN FOR FOOD & DRINKS

| Low Fat Breakfast | Morning Snack | Low Fat Lunch | Afternoon Snack | Low Fat Evening Meal | Evening Snack (Optional) | 2-3 Units |

You could painstakingly write down all of this. Or you could record a number into a box and this is where your IntaShape score comes in. Your score card is at the heart of this plan and only takes a few seconds each day to complete. Your score card has two sections and is located on the back of the last page of this book.

The first section is for you to record your daily score for food and drinks and is very easy to use. If you followed the plan to the letter on Day 1, then all you have to do is write the number 5 in the Day 1 box in the Food & Drinks Section of your score card.

FOOD & DRINKS SECTION

	Day 1	Day 2	Day 3	Day 4	Day 5	Day 6	Day 7	FOOD & DRINK SCORE
Week 1	5 +	+	+	+	+	+	=	

| Low Fat Breakfast | Morning Snack | Low Fat Lunch | Afternoon Snack | Low Fat Evening Meal | Evening Snack (Optional) | 2-3 Units |

If you followed the plan to the letter every day you would score 5 points every day as follows:

Monday: Followed the plan and scored 5 points.

Tuesday: Followed the plan and scored 5 points.

Wednesday: Followed the plan and scored 5 points.

Thursday: Followed the plan and scored 5 points.

Friday: Followed the plan and scored 5 points.

Saturday: Followed the plan and scored 5 points.

Sunday: Followed the plan and scored 5 points.

All you have to do at the end of the day is to write the number 5 in each box in the Food & Drinks Section of your Score Card.

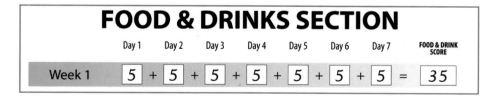

FOOD & DRINKS SECTION

	Day 1	Day 2	Day 3	Day 4	Day 5	Day 6	Day 7	FOOD & DRINK SCORE
Week 1	5	+ 5	+ 5	+ 5	+ 5	+ 5	+ 5 =	35

At the end of the week you add up your daily scores and insert this number into the last box marked Food & Drink Score. This would be a maximum of 35 points.

REAL LIFE DAYS

You are not expected to go through the next six weeks scoring **5** points every day. Do not think that you are a failure because you did not score 5 points on any one day!

There will be days when scoring 5 points a day will be impossible. All you do on those days is score your day differently. **4, 3, 2, 1, 0** are also scores you can record following this plan.

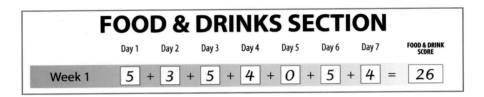

Look to score higher through the week and you can be a bit more relaxed at the weekend. In this example Day 5 (Friday) was a really bad day, so a 0 is inserted for Day 5. It's as easy as that.

Consequently the weekly score for Food & Drinks has been reduced from a possible 35 down to 26. You can still lose inches with a score of 26 for Food & Drinks.

You will really only know how well your day has been and what your final score will be after your last meal or drink. Following the plan and making good choices means that you will keep all your points and score a maximum of 5 points. You only lose points when you stray from the best choices.

The easiest way to do this is to start each day with 5 points and by making the best choices you hold onto all 5 points. When it is not possible to make the best choices, then, you start to deduct points from your score of 5 points. The next few pages explain how you lose these points.

MEALS

The higher the total fat content of each meal is
above 10 grams of fat then the more points you lose for that meal.

YOU START EACH DAY WITH 5 POINTS...

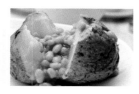

• Lose 0 points for any meal up to 10 grams of fat.

• Lose 1 point for each meal between 11-19 grams of fat.

• Lose 2 points for each meal between 20-29 grams of fat.

• Lose 3 points for each meal between 30-39 grams of fat.

• Lose 4 points for each meal between 40-49 grams of fat.

• Lose all 5 points for any meal with 50 or more grams of fat.

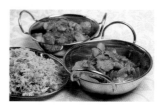

SNACKS

The higher the total fat content of each snack is above 10 grams of fat then the more points you lose for that snack.

YOU START EACH DAY WITH 5 POINTS...

- Lose 0 points for a mid-morning fresh fruit snack.

- Lose 0 points for a mid-afternoon fresh fruit snack.

- Lose 0 points for any evening snack up to 10 grams of fat.

- Lose 1 point for each snack between 11-19 grams of fat.

- Lose 2 points for each snack between 20-29 grams of fat.

- Lose 3 points for each snack between 30-39 grams of fat.

- Lose 4 points for each snack between 40-49 grams of fat.

- Lose all 5 points for any snack with 50 or more grams of fat.

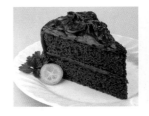

ALCOHOLIC DRINKS

The more units of alcohol that you drink above the daily recommendations then the more points you lose.

YOU START EACH DAY WITH 5 POINTS...

DAILY RECOMMENDED INTAKE

WOMEN: No more than 2 units of alcohol per day.

MEN: No more than 3 units of alcohol per day.

Lose 1 point for every 2 units of alcohol you drink each day above these daily recommendations.

BONUS DAYS
Fridays & Saturdays

You can have an additional 2 units of alcohol on both of these days without losing any points.

If you do drink alcohol then plan to have one to two days a week that are alcohol free.

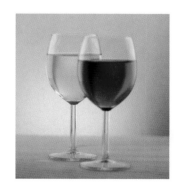

EXAMPLES OF SCORING
FOOD & DRINKS
FROM
MONDAY - SUNDAY

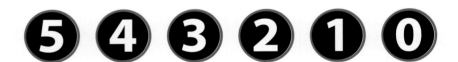

EXAMPLES OF SCORING

DAY 1 – MONDAY
YOU START EACH DAY WITH 5 POINTS

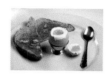

BREAKFAST
Up to 10 grams of fat.
Lose 0 points.

MORNING SNACK
Fresh fruit.
Lose 0 points.

LUNCH
Up to 10 grams of fat.
Lose 0 points.

AFTERNOON SNACK
Fresh fruit.
Lose 0 points.

EARLY EVENING SNACK
Up to 10 grams of fat.
Lose 0 points.

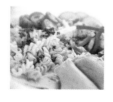

EVENING MEAL
Up to 10 grams of fat.
Lose 0 points.

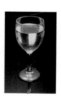

ALCOHOL
2 units.
Lose 0 points.

You started with 5 points and still have 5 points left at the end of the day.
Record 5 in Day 1 of your score card.

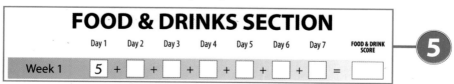

FOOD & DRINKS SECTION

	Day 1	Day 2	Day 3	Day 4	Day 5	Day 6	Day 7	FOOD & DRINK SCORE	
Week 1	5	+	+	+	+	+	+	=	5

EXAMPLES OF SCORING

DAY 2 – TUESDAY
YOU START EACH DAY WITH 5 POINTS

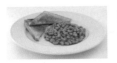 **BREAKFAST**
Up to 10 grams of fat.
Lose 0 points.

 MORNING SNACK
20-29g of fat.
Lose 0 points.

 LUNCH
Up to 10 grams of fat.
Lose 0 points.
Lose 0 points.

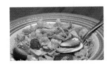 **AFTERNOON SNACK**
Fresh fruit.

 EARLY EVENING SNACK
Up to 10 grams of fat.
Lose 0 points.

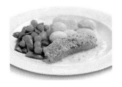 **EVENING MEAL**
Up to 10 grams of fat.
Lose 0 points.

 ALCOHOL
2 units.
Lose 0 points.

You started with 5 points, 2 points deducted for the morning snack leaving you with 3 points. Record 3 in Day 2 of your score card.

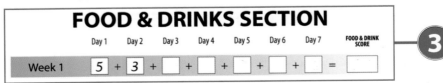

FOOD & DRINKS SECTION

	Day 1	Day 2	Day 3	Day 4	Day 5	Day 6	Day 7	FOOD & DRINK SCORE
Week 1	5 +	3 +	+	+	+	+	+	=

3

EXAMPLES OF SCORING

DAY 3 – WEDNESDAY
YOU START EACH DAY WITH 5 POINTS

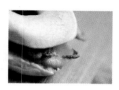

BREAKFAST
Up to 10 grams of fat.
Lose 0 points.

MORNING SNACK
Fresh fruit.
Lose 0 points.

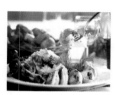

LUNCH
Up to 10 grams of fat.
Lose 0 points.

AFTERNOON SNACK
Fresh fruit.
Lose 0 points.

EARLY EVENING SNACK
Up to 10 grams of fat.
Lose 0 points.

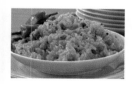

EVENING MEAL
Up to 10 grams of fat.
Lose 0 points.

ALCOHOL
0 units.
Lose 0 points.

*You started with 5 points and still have 5 points left at the end of the day.
Record 5 in Day 3 of your score card.*

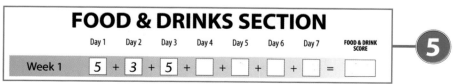

FOOD & DRINKS SECTION

	Day 1	Day 2	Day 3	Day 4	Day 5	Day 6	Day 7	FOOD & DRINK SCORE
Week 1	5 +	3 +	5 +	+	+	+	=	

5

EXAMPLES OF SCORING

DAY 4 – THURSDAY
YOU START EACH DAY WITH 5 POINTS

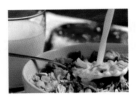

BREAKFAST
Up to 10 grams of fat.
Lose 0 points.

MORNING SNACK
Fresh fruit.
Lose 0 points.

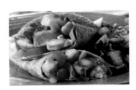

LUNCH
Up to 10 grams of fat.
Lose 0 points.

AFTERNOON SNACK
Fresh fruit.
Lose 0 points.

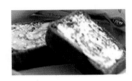

EARLY EVENING SNACK
Up to 10 grams of fat.
Lose 0 points.

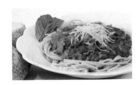

EVENING MEAL
11-19 grams of fat.
Lose 1 point.

ALCOHOL
2 units.
Lose 0 points.

*You started with 5 points,
1 point deducted for the evening meal leaving you with 4 points.
Record 4 in Day 4 of your score card.*

FOOD & DRINKS SECTION

	Day 1	Day 2	Day 3	Day 4	Day 5	Day 6	Day 7	FOOD & DRINK SCORE
Week 1	5 +	3 +	5 +	4 +	+	+	=	

4

EXAMPLES OF SCORING

DAY 5 – FRIDAY
YOU START EACH DAY WITH 5 POINTS

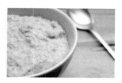

BREAKFAST
Up to 10 grams of fat.
Lose 0 points.

MORNING SNACK
Fresh fruit.
Lose 0 points.

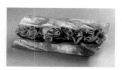

LUNCH
Up to 10 grams of fat.
Lose 0 points.

AFTERNOON SNACK
Fresh fruit.
Lose 0 points.

EARLY EVENING SNACK
Up to 10 grams of fat.
Lose 0 points.

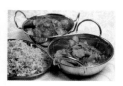

EVENING MEAL
50 grams or more.
Lose 5 points.

ALCOHOL
4 units.
Lose 0 points.

*You started with 5 points and lost all 5 points through the evening meal.
Record 0 in Day 5 of your score card.*

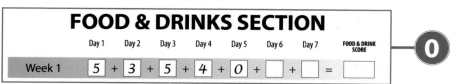

FOOD & DRINKS SECTION

	Day 1	Day 2	Day 3	Day 4	Day 5	Day 6	Day 7	FOOD & DRINK SCORE	
Week 1	5 +	3 +	5 +	4 +	0 +	+	=		0

EXAMPLES OF SCORING

DAY 6 – SATURDAY
YOU START EACH DAY WITH 5 POINTS

 BREAKFAST
Up to 10 grams of fat.
Lose 0 points.

 MORNING SNACK
Fresh orange.
Lose 0 points.

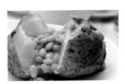 **LUNCH**
Up to 10 grams of fat.
Lose 0 points.

 AFTERNOON SNACK
Fresh fruit.
Lose 0 points.

EARLY EVENING SNACK
None.
Lose 0 points.

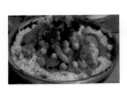 **EVENING MEAL**
Up to 10 grams of fat.
Lose 0 points.

 ALCOHOL
4 units.
Lose 0 points.

You started with 5 points and lost no points.
Record 5 in Day 6 of your score card.

FOOD & DRINKS SECTION

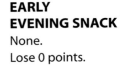

	Day 1	Day 2	Day 3	Day 4	Day 5	Day 6	Day 7	FOOD & DRINK SCORE
Week 1	5 +	3 +	5 +	4 +	0 +	5 +		=

5

DAY 7 – SUNDAY
YOU START EACH DAY WITH 5 POINTS

BREAKFAST
Up to 10 grams of fat.
Lose 0 points.

MORNING SNACK
Fresh fruit.
Lose 0 points.

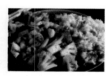

LUNCH
Up to 10 grams of fat.
Lose 0 points.

AFTERNOON SNACK
Fresh fruit.
Lose 0 points.

EARLY EVENING SNACK
None.
Lose 0 points.

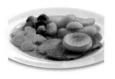

EVENING MEAL
11-19 grams of fat.
Lose 1 point.

ALCOHOL
0 units.
Lose 0 points.

You started with 5 points, 1 point lost through the evening meal.
Record 4 in Day 7 of your score card.
Food & Drink Score for Week 1 came to 26 points.

FOOD & DRINKS SECTION

	Day 1	Day 2	Day 3	Day 4	Day 5	Day 6	Day 7	FOOD & DRINK SCORE
Week 1	5	+ 3	+ 5	+ 4	+ 0	+ 5	+ 4	= 26

4

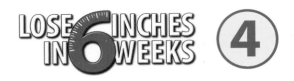

GET ACTIVE

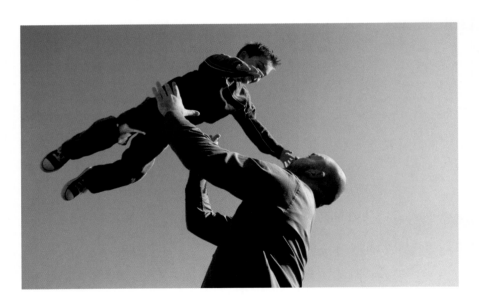

ACTIVITIES

This section is to introduce you to how you score points for being active. Activities include walking, brisk walking, cycling, swimming, gym, exercise classes all count. Although you score the same amount of points for exercise as you do for walking, you will be using more calories though exercise and improving your fitness at the same time.

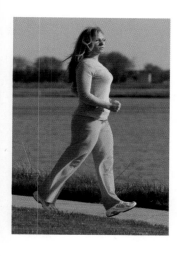

- **10 minutes of physical activity score 1 point**

- **20 minutes of physical activity score 2 points**

- **30 minutes of physical activity score 3 points**

- **40 minutes of physical activity score 4 points**

- **50 minutes of physical activity score 5 points**

The most you can score on any day for activity is 5 points. However, the more physically active you are, then the more calories will be used as energy.

ACTIVITIES & SCORING VALUES

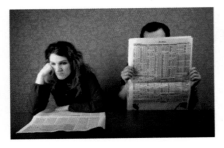

SITTING
Sitting is a very low calorie activity.
You score 0 points.

WALKING
Walking uses twice as many calories than sitting.
You score 1 point for every 10 minutes of walking.
You can score up to 5 points for a total of 50 minutes.

BRISK WALKING
Brisk walking uses three times as many calories than sitting.
You score 1 point for every 10 minutes of brisk walking.
You can score up to 5 points for a total of 50 minutes.

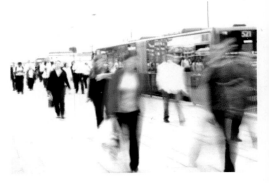

EXERCISE
Exercise can use up to four times as many calories as sitting.
You score 1 point for every 10 minutes of exercise.
You can score up to 5 points for a total of 50 minutes.

There are 168 hours in a week, most of these are spent either sitting or laying down. Even if you workout for three hours a week, it's what you do during the remaining 165 hours that makes a difference. The scoring system caters for activities both inside and outside a gym.

EXAMPLES OF SCORING ACTIVITY

The Activity Section of your score card is your guide to how active you are each day and the number of calories you will have lost as energy.

DAY 1

Let's say on your first day of following the plan you did a total of 40 minutes walking during the whole day then you record 4 in the box for Day 1.

DAY 2

On your second day you did 30 minutes swimming. Plus a total of 20 minutes walking spread across the day then you record 5 in the box for Day 2.

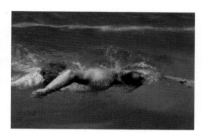

DAY 3

On your third day you did 20 minutes walking in the morning and another 20 minutes walking at lunchtime then you record 4 in the box for Day 3.

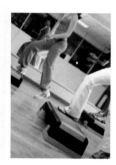

DAY 4

On your fourth day you did a 50 minute exercise workout, then you record 5 in the box for Day 4.

ACTIVITY SECTION

	Day 1	Day 2	Day 3	Day 4	Day 5	Day 6	Day 7	ACTIVITY SCORE	COMBINED SCORE
Week 1	4 +	5 +	4 +	5 +	+	+	=		

EXAMPLES OF SCORING ACTIVITY

DAY 5

On your fifth day you did 30 minutes brisk walking.
You record 3 in the box for Day 5.

DAY 6

On your sixth day you did some cycling and some
walking that came to a combined total of 60
minutes. You record 5 in the box for Day 6 as this
is the most you can score on any one day. You will
see the benefits of the extra minutes at the end of
the 6 weeks!

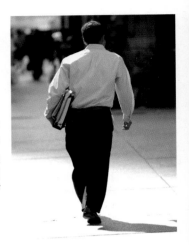

DAY 7

On your seventh day you did 30 minutes walking. You record 3 in the box for
Day 7. You then add up your total score for the week and record that in the box
for Activity Score. In this example it came to 29.

ACTIVITY SECTION

	Day 1		Day 2		Day 3		Day 4		Day 5		Day 6		Day 7		ACTIVITY SCORE	COMBINED SCORE
Week 1	4	+	5	+	4	+	5	+	3	+	5	+	3	=	29	

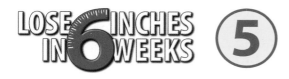

HOW TO
LOSE 6 INCHES
IN 6 WEEKS

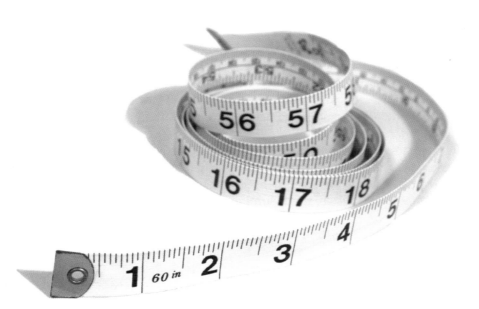

YOUR MOTIVATIONAL HELPER

This is where your score card becomes a motivational helper. At the end of each week you take the weekly score for Food & Drinks (26), and add this to the weekly score for Activity (29). This gives you a weekly total of 55 points.

FOOD & DRINKS SECTION

	Day 1	Day 2	Day 3	Day 4	Day 5	Day 6	Day 7	FOOD & DRINK SCORE
Week 1	5 +	3 +	5 +	4 +	0 +	5 +	4 =	26

ACTIVITY SECTION

	Day 1	Day 2	Day 3	Day 4	Day 5	Day 6	Day 7	ACTIVITY SCORE	COMBINED SCORE
Week 1	4 +	5 +	4 +	5 +	3 +	5 +	3 =	29	55

You carry on completing your score card for the next 6 weeks. Your score card is located on the back of the last page of this book. To lose 6 inches in 6 weeks you need to average a particular score each week to be sure of success. This weekly average score is based on a number of personal factors, some you can influence, others you cannot. The main one, which you cannot influence, is your height.

The taller you are, in general terms, the more calories your body should use as energy each day. As previously discussed, men can use more calories each day than women can. This is because men, as a general rule, tend to be taller and have more lean mass (muscle) than women.

When you come to measure your body at the start and again after 6 weeks, men have seven areas to measure, while women have eight areas. The result is that both can use the same scale to lose 6 inches in 6 weeks.

WHAT YOU HAVE TO DO TO LOSE 6 INCHES IN 6 WEEKS

1. Record your scores each day for Food & Drinks and for Activity for the next 6 weeks onto your score card which is located on the back of the last page of this book.

FOOD & DRINKS SECTION

	Day 1	Day 2	Day 3	Day 4	Day 5	Day 6	Day 7	FOOD & DRINK SCORE
Week 1	5 +	3 +	5 +	4 +	0 +	5 +	4 =	26
Week 2	5 +	5 +	2 +	5 +	5 +	2 +	2 =	26
Week 3	5 +	4 +	4 +	4 +	5 +	0 +	0 =	22
Week 4	5 +	4 +	4 +	4 +	5 +	4 +	4 =	30
Week 5	5 +	4 +	3 +	5 +	3 +	2 +	0 =	22
Week 6	5 +	5 +	4 +	4 +	5 +	3 +	0 =	26

ACTIVITY SECTION

	Day 1	Day 2	Day 3	Day 4	Day 5	Day 6	Day 7	ACTIVITY SCORE	COMBINED SCORE
Week 1	4 +	5 +	4 +	5 +	3 +	5 +	3 =	29	55
Week 2	3 +	5 +	4 +	4 +	4 +	5 +	5 =	30	56
Week 3	4 +	4 +	5 +	4 +	3 +	5 +	5 =	30	52
Week 4	5 +	3 +	5 +	4 +	5 +	5 +	1 =	28	58
Week 5	5 +	5 +	5 +	5 +	4 +	5 +	5 =	34	56
Week 6	4 +	4 +	4 +	4 +	4 +	4 +	4 =	28	54

2. On completion of the 6 weeks add up your weekly combined totals and divide this number by six to give you your weekly average for the six weeks.

3. To lose 6 inches you need to achieve the following average score over the 6 weeks, which is based on your height.

THE INTASHAPE INCH LOSS PLAN

HEIGHT	AVERAGE WEEKLY SCORE TO LOSE 6 INCHES IN 6 WEEKS
Taller than 184cm Taller than 6ft:	An average of at least 48 points.
171cm -184cm 5ft 7in to 6ft:	An average of at least 50 points.
164cm – 171cm 5ft 4in to 5ft 7in:	An average of at least 52 points.
155cm – 164cm 5ft 1in to 5ft 4in:	An average of at least 54 points.
Smaller than 155cm Smaller than 5ft 1in:	An average of at least 56 points.

MEASUREMENTS

The measurements are based on the circumference measurements from eight body areas for women and seven for men. Men should not measure the area of the hips (shown as area 3 below). The diagram below shows the areas of your body that you should measure. If you need to weigh yourself then this has also been included.

To measure yourself you will need a normal tape measure. Always try to use the same tape measure as they do differ. You can record your measurements in either centimetres (CM) or in inches.

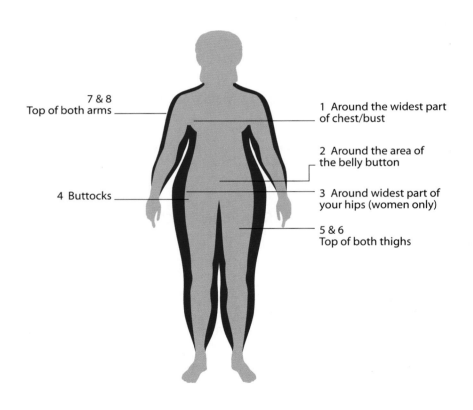

7 & 8
Top of both arms

1 Around the widest part of chest/bust

2 Around the area of the belly button

4 Buttocks

3 Around widest part of your hips (women only)

5 & 6
Top of both thighs

EXAMPLE OF MEASUREMENTS

No	Body Area	Dates 14/05/07 Starting Measurements	23/06/07 Measurements After 6 Weeks	Cm/Inches Lost
1	Chest/Bust	94cm	92cm	2cm
2	Waist	91.5cm	87cm	4.5cm
3	Hips (Women only)	100cm	97cm	3cm
4	Buttocks	107cm	103cm	4cm
5	Right Thigh	65cm	63.5cm	1.5cm
6	Left Thigh	65cm	63.5cm	1.5cm
7	Right Arm	34cm	33cm	1cm
8	Left Arm	34cm	33cm	1cm
	Total inches/centimetres lost (To convert centimetres to inches you divide by 2.5)			18.5cm 7.5inches
	Weight	150 pounds	143 pounds	7 pounds

RECORD YOUR MEASUREMENTS

No	Body Area	Dates Starting Measurements	Measurements After 6 Weeks	Cm/Inches Lost
1	Chest/Bust			
2	Waist			
3	Hips (Women only)			
4	Buttocks			
5	Right Thigh			
6	Left Thigh			
7	Right Arm			
8	Left Arm			
	Total inches/centimetres lost			
	Weight			

DAY 1 - BREAKFAST

This is to guide you through your first day to help you come to terms with just how easy it is to use your score card. Starting with scoring the Food & Drinks section.

Remember that you start each day with 5 points, with the aim of holding onto as many of these 5 points as you can.

BREAKFAST
(Breaking the fast)

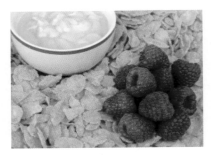

Breakfast is arguably the most important meal of the day. Get breakfast right and you start the day well. Go to the Easy Low-Fat Meals section (starts on page 90) of this book and select any one of the breakfast examples to keep your 5 points. Alternatively, you can make up your own breakfast with up to 10 grams of fat and you still keep your 5 points.

*Select any breakfast with a higher fat content
and you deduct points as follows...*

- **Lose 1 point for any breakfast between 11-19 grams of fat.**

- **Lose 2 points for any breakfast between 20-29 grams of fat.**

- **Lose 3 points for any breakfast between 30-39 grams of fat.**

- **Lose 4 points for any breakfast between 40-49 grams of fat.**

- **Lose all 5 points for any breakfast with 50 or more grams of fat.**

Please record the number of points you still have left after breakfast in this box.

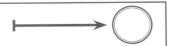

DAY 1 - MID-MORNING SNACK

Even though you have had breakfast, by around mid-morning your energy levels will begin to drop. A mid-morning snack will top up your energy levels and keep you going until lunch. Undoubtedly, the healthiest mid-morning snack is fresh fruit. Fresh fruit is a good source of antioxidants and provides water and fibre. If you miss a mid-morning fresh fruit snack then you deduct 1 point.

- **1 small banana**

- **1 pear**

- **1 apple**

- **2 plums**

- **1 orange**

- **1 peach**

- **1 handful of soft fruit**

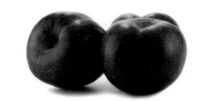

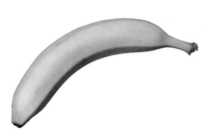

Please record the number of points you still have left after your mid-morning snack in this box.

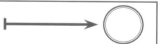

Note...
At the weekend you may not need a mid-morning snack as breakfast is usually a bit later in the morning. If this is the case, then even if you do not have a mid-morning snack, you do not lose any points.

DAY 1 - LUNCH

Lunch is the meal that sets you up to get you through the most of the afternoon.

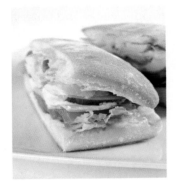

Again go to the Easy Low-Fat Meals section (starts on page 90) of this book and select any one of the example meals to keep your 5 points.

Alternatively, you can make up your own lunch with up to 10 grams of fat and you still keep your 5 points.

Select any lunch with a higher fat content and you deduct points as follows...

- **Lose 1 point for any meal between 11-19 grams of fat.**
- **Lose 2 points for any meal between 20-29 grams of fat.**
- **Lose 3 points for any meal between 30-39 grams of fat.**
- **Lose 4 points for any meal between 40-49 grams of fat.**
- **Lose all 5 points for any meal with 50 or more grams of fat.**

Please record the number of points you still have left after lunch in this box.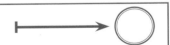

DAY 1 - MID-AFTERNOON SNACK

A mid-afternoon snack will top up your energy levels and keep you going during the later part of the afternoon. Like your mid-morning snack, fresh fruit is your best choice. If you miss a mid-afternoon fresh fruit snack then you deduct 1 point.

1 apple

1 pear

1 small banana

2 plums

1 orange

1 peach

1 handful of soft fruit

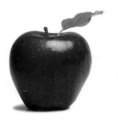

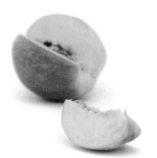

Please record the number of points you still have left after your mid-afternoon snack in this box.

DAY 1 - EVENING MEAL

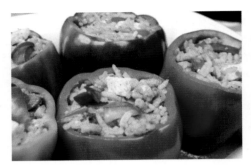

Once more go to the Easy Low-Fat Meals section (starts on page 90) of this book and select any one of the example meals to keep your 5 points. Alternatively, you can make up your own evening meal with up to 10 grams of fat and you still keep your 5 points.

Select any meal with a higher fat content and you deduct points as follows...

- **Lose 1 point for any meal between 11-19 grams of fat**
- **Lose 2 points for any meal between 20-29 grams of fat**
- **Lose 3 points for any meal between 30-39 grams of fat**
- **Lose 4 points for any meal between 40-49 grams of fat**
- **Lose all 5 points for any meal with 50 or more grams of fat**

Please record the number of points you still have left after your evening meal in this box.

DAY 1 - EVENING SNACK

The time you have your evening meal is your guide to when you should have an evening snack. Your evening snack is optional and you do not lot lose any points if you feel you do not need this snack.

If you're planning to have your evening meal after 7pm then you may benefit from enjoying an early evening snack around 5pm. If you have an early evening meal and you still feel hungry later then have your snack later. Examples of good evening snacks are as follows.

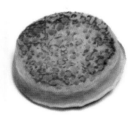

1 toasted crumpet with 1 tsp of low fat spread.

1 pot of low fat yogurt with a few nuts.

1 slice of malt loaf with low fat spread.

Small bag of pretzels (60g).

2 crispbreads with 2tbsp of low fat cottage cheese.

1 low fat cereal bar.

1 fruit smoothie (250g).

Small bowl (25g) of cereal with 150ml semi-skimmed milk and some chopped fruit.

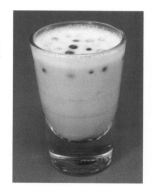

1 low fat muffin.

1 slice wholemeal toast with 2tsp of jam or honey.

DAY 1 - EVENING SNACK

Choose any evening snack with more than 10 grams of fat and you lose points as follows.

- Lose 1 point for any snack between 11-19 grams of fat.

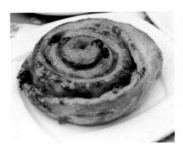

- Lose 2 points for any meal between 20-29 grams of fat.

- Lose 3 points for any meal between 30-39 grams of fat.

- Lose 4 points for any meal between 40-49 grams of fat.

- Lose all 5 points for any meal with 50 or more grams of fat.

Please record the number of points you still have left after your evening snack in this box. ⟶ ◯

Note...
You also lose the same number of points if you have any of these as a mid-morning or mid-afternoon snack.

DAY 1 - ALCOHOL

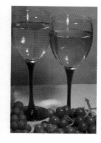

If you do drink alcohol, then please use the table below to score your alcohol intake.

ALCOHOL	Women Points Lost	Men Points Lost
Up to 2 units/day	0	0
Up to 3 units/day	1	0
4 units/day	2	1
6 units/day	3	2
8 units/day	4	3
10 units/day	5	4
11 units/day		5

Plan to have at least two days a week that are alcohol free. You can have an additional two units on Fridays & Saturdays without losing any points.

Please record the number of points you still have left after you take into consideration any alcohol you consumed today in this box. ⟶ ◯

This is your score for Food & Drinks for today.
Record this number onto Day 1 of your score card,
which is on the back of the last page of this book.

FOOD & DRINKS SECTION

	Day 1	Day 2	Day 3	Day 4	Day 5	Day 6	Day 7	FOOD & DRINK SCORE
Week 1	☐ +	☐ +	☐ +	☐ +	☐ +	☐ +	☐ =	☐

DAY 1 - ACTIVITY

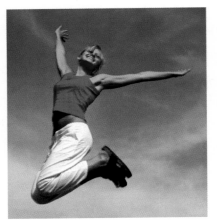

This is to guide you through your first day on scoring your Activity. Unlike the Food & Drinks section where you start each day with 5 and try to hold on to as many points as you can. You start each day with 0 points and build up to a maximum of 5 points each day through various physical activities as follows.

ACTIVITY	TIME	POINTS SCORED
Walking or Exercise	10 minutes	1 point
Walking or Exercise	20 minutes	2 points
Walking or Exercise	30 minutes	3 points
Walking or Exercise	40 minutes	4 points
Walking or Exercise	50 + minutes	5 points

(0) ## TIME SEGMENTS

This page has your day broken down into different time segments. After each time segment record any activity points you achieved during that period. Breaking your day down into the different time segments gives you the opportunity to see the times of the day when you are physically active and when you are not. You start each day with 0 points.

( ) ## FIRST THING IN THE MORNING TO YOUR MID-MORNING BREAK

If you have been physically active for at least 10 minutes during this period then record the appropriate number in this box. Can you make improvements here?

( ) ## MID-MORNING BREAK UNTIL LUNCHTIME

If you have been physically active for at least 10 minutes during this period then record the appropriate number in this box. Could you be more active at this time?

( ) ## LUNCH UNTIL LATE AFTERNOON (5pm)

If you have been physically active for at least 10 minutes during this period then record the appropriate number in this box. Is this an area of opportunity for you?

( ) ## THE EVENING

If you have been physically active for at least 10 minutes during this period then record the appropriate number in this box. How can you be more active here?

( ) ## ACTIVITY SCORE

Total up the number of activity points that you have scored today and record the total in this box. Remember that the most you can record in this box is 5 points.

This is your score for Activity for today.
Record this number onto Day 1 of your score card.

ACTIVITY SECTION

	Day 1		Day 2		Day 3		Day 4		Day 5		Day 6		Day 7		ACTIVITY SCORE	COMBINED SCORE
Week 1	☐	+	☐	+	☐	+	☐	+	☐	+	☐	+	☐	=	☐	☐

SCORING THE REST OF WEEK 1

The next few pages give you the opportunity to continue to score your day in this way for the rest of the week. At the end of each day your just transfer your scores onto your score card.

On completion of your first week you can then record your scores at the end of each day directly onto your score card.

FOOD & DRINKS SECTION

	Day 1		Day 2		Day 3		Day 4		Day 5		Day 6		Day 7		FOOD & DRINK SCORE
Week 1		+		+		+		+		+		+		=	
Week 2		+		+		+		+		+		+		=	
Week 3		+		+		+		+		+		+		=	
Week 4		+		+		+		+		+		+		=	
Week 5		+		+		+		+		+		+		=	
Week 6		+		+		+		+		+		+		=	

ACTIVITY SECTION

	Day 1		Day 2		Day 3		Day 4		Day 5		Day 6		Day 7		ACTIVITY SCORE	COMBINED SCORE
Week 1		+		+		+		+		+		+		=		
Week 2		+		+		+		+		+		+		=		
Week 3		+		+		+		+		+		+		=		
Week 4		+		+		+		+		+		+		=		
Week 5		+		+		+		+		+		+		=		
Week 6		+		+		+		+		+		+		=		

WEEK 1
DAY 2 - FOOD & DRINKS

5 **YOU START WITH 5 POINTS**

○ BREAKFAST

○ MID-MORNING SNACK

○ LUNCH

○ MID-AFTERNOON SNACK

○ EVENING MEAL

○ EVENING SNACK

○ **ALCOHOL** (Please deduct any points for alcohol and record this number onto your score card.)

DAY 2 - ACTIVITY

0 **YOU START WITH ZERO POINTS**

○ FIRST THING IN THE MORNING TO YOUR MID-MORNING BREAK

○ MID-MORNING BREAK UNTIL LUNCHTIME

○ LUNCH UNTIL LATE AFTERNOON (5pm)

○ THE EVENING

○ **ACTIVITY SCORE** (Record this number onto your score card)

WEEK 1
DAY 3 - FOOD & DRINKS

(5) **YOU START WITH 5 POINTS**

◯ BREAKFAST

◯ MID-MORNING SNACK

◯ LUNCH

◯ MID-AFTERNOON SNACK

◯ EVENING MEAL

◯ EVENING SNACK

◯ **ALCOHOL** (Please deduct any points for alcohol and record this number onto your score card.)

DAY 3 - ACTIVITY

(0) **YOU START WITH ZERO POINTS**

◯ FIRST THING IN THE MORNING TO YOUR MID-MORNING BREAK

◯ MID-MORNING BREAK UNTIL LUNCHTIME

◯ LUNCH UNTIL LATE AFTERNOON (5pm)

◯ THE EVENING

◯ **ACTIVITY SCORE** (Record this number onto your score card)

WEEK 1
DAY 4 - FOOD & DRINKS

5 **YOU START WITH 5 POINTS**

◯ BREAKFAST

◯ MID-MORNING SNACK

◯ LUNCH

◯ MID-AFTERNOON SNACK

◯ EVENING MEAL

◯ EVENING SNACK

◯ **ALCOHOL** (Please deduct any points for alcohol and record this number onto your score card.)

DAY 4 - ACTIVITY

0 **YOU START WITH ZERO POINTS**

◯ FIRST THING IN THE MORNING TO YOUR MID-MORNING BREAK

◯ MID-MORNING BREAK UNTIL LUNCHTIME

◯ LUNCH UNTIL LATE AFTERNOON (5pm)

◯ THE EVENING

◯ **ACTIVITY SCORE** (Record this number onto your score card)

WEEK 1
DAY 5 - FOOD & DRINKS

(5) **YOU START WITH 5 POINTS**

◯ BREAKFAST

◯ MID-MORNING SNACK

◯ LUNCH

◯ MID-AFTERNOON SNACK

◯ EVENING MEAL

◯ EVENING SNACK

◯ **ALCOHOL** (Please deduct any points for alcohol and record this number onto your score card.)

DAY 5 - ACTIVITY

(0) **YOU START WITH ZERO POINTS**

◯ FIRST THING IN THE MORNING TO YOUR MID-MORNING BREAK

◯ MID-MORNING BREAK UNTIL LUNCHTIME

◯ LUNCH UNTIL LATE AFTERNOON (5pm)

◯ THE EVENING

◯ **ACTIVITY SCORE** (Record this number onto your score card)

WEEK 1
DAY 6 - FOOD & DRINKS

5 **YOU START WITH 5 POINTS**

○ BREAKFAST

○ MID-MORNING SNACK

○ LUNCH

○ MID-AFTERNOON SNACK

○ EVENING MEAL

○ EVENING SNACK

○ **ALCOHOL** (Please deduct any points for alcohol and record this number onto your score card.)

DAY 6 - ACTIVITY

0 **YOU START WITH ZERO POINTS**

○ FIRST THING IN THE MORNING TO YOUR MID-MORNING BREAK

○ MID-MORNING BREAK UNTIL LUNCHTIME

○ LUNCH UNTIL LATE AFTERNOON (5pm)

○ THE EVENING

○ **ACTIVITY SCORE** (Record this number onto your score card)

WEEK 1
DAY 7 - FOOD & DRINKS

(5) **YOU START WITH 5 POINTS**

◯ BREAKFAST

◯ MID-MORNING SNACK

◯ LUNCH

◯ MID-AFTERNOON SNACK

◯ EVENING MEAL

◯ EVENING SNACK

◯ **ALCOHOL** (Please deduct any points for alcohol and record this number onto your score card.)

DAY 7 - ACTIVITY

(0) **YOU START WITH ZERO POINTS**

◯ FIRST THING IN THE MORNING
TO YOUR MID-MORNING BREAK

◯ MID-MORNING BREAK UNTIL LUNCHTIME

◯ LUNCH UNTIL LATE AFTERNOON (5pm)

◯ THE EVENING

◯ **ACTIVITY SCORE** (Record this number onto your score card)

HOW MANY INCHES HAVE YOU LOST?

At the end of the 6 weeks your score card will be completed.

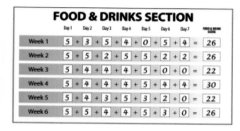

FOOD & DRINKS SECTION

	Day 1	Day 2	Day 3	Day 4	Day 5	Day 6	Day 7	FOOD & DRINK SCORE
Week 1	5 +	3 +	5 +	4 +	0 +	5 +	4 =	26
Week 2	5 +	5 +	2 +	5 +	5 +	2 +	2 =	26
Week 3	5 +	4 +	4 +	4 +	5 +	0 +	0 =	22
Week 4	5 +	4 +	4 +	4 +	5 +	4 +	4 =	30
Week 5	5 +	4 +	3 +	5 +	3 +	2 +	0 =	22
Week 6	5 +	5 +	4 +	4 +	5 +	3 +	0 =	26

ACTIVITY SECTION

	Day 1	Day 2	Day 3	Day 4	Day 5	Day 6	Day 7	ACTIVITY SCORE	COMBINED SCORE
Week 1	4 +	5 +	4 +	5 +	3 +	5 +	3 =	29	55
Week 2	3 +	5 +	4 +	4 +	4 +	5 +	5 =	30	56
Week 3	4 +	4 +	5 +	4 +	3 +	5 +	5 =	30	52
Week 4	5 +	3 +	5 +	4 +	5 +	5 +	1 =	28	58
Week 5	5 +	5 +	5 +	5 +	4 +	5 +	5 =	34	56
Week 6	4 +	4 +	4 +	4 +	4 +	4 +	4 =	28	54

Add up your weekly combined totals and divide this number by six to give you your weekly average for the six weeks. In the example above the total score came to 331 points. Divide 331 by 6 and the weekly average comes to 55.

Then compare your total loss in inches to the average based on your height and see how well you have done.

THE INTASHAPE INCH LOSS PLAN

HEIGHT	AVERAGE WEEKLY SCORE TO LOSE 6 INCHES IN 6 WEEKS
Taller than 184cm Taller than 6ft	An average of at least 48 points
171cm -184cm 5ft 7in to 6ft	An average of at least 50 points
164cm – 171cm 5ft 4in to 5ft 7in	An average of at least 52 points
155cm – 164cm 5ft 1in to 5ft 4in	An average of at least 54 points
Smaller than 155cm Smaller than 5ft 1in	An average of at least 56 points

Do not be surprised if at the end of 6 weeks you have lost more than 6 inches.

A FEW TIPS

SCORING

Unless you put on an electronic device that accurately measures the amount of calories you use up each day, scoring your activity will always be a personal decision. There will be occasions when your activity will not fall into nice little 10 minute slots. An example of this is if you are looking after young children and are continually on the go and moving around, or, you have a physically active job.

If you have days where you are continuously moving around, then look to score between one to five points on these days. This is your call, because only you will know how active you have been.

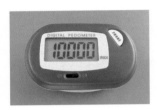

USE A PEDOMETER

A pedometer is a great way to measure your daily activity levels. A pedometer measures the number of steps you do. Once you have set up your pedometer to measure your steps then use the following guide to score the number of steps you do each day.

Number of Steps	Activity Points
2,000 steps	1 point
4,000 steps	2 points
6,000 steps	3 points
8,000 steps	4 points
10,000+ steps	5 points

RECRUIT A BUDDY

Get a friend to start with you. You can measure each other at the beginning of the plan and at the end of 6 weeks. Look to plan the week ahead with your friend, especially for activities like going out for walks, swimming, cycling or even joining a gym. At the end of each week you can plan to sit down together and discuss how your week has been. Check with each other that your scores are correct and look to set new weekly scores together.

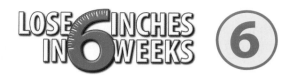

THE SILENT
ASSASSIN

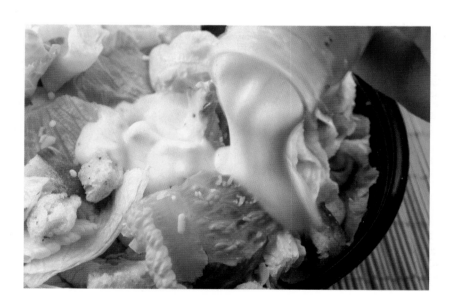

FAT

There is one incredibly subtle force that can play a major role in destroying your shape on the outside, and can kill you from the inside. Yet used in the right way can improve your health and your shape. That subtle force is called fat.

If not controlled, fat will slowly and silently, inch by inch, over the years, creep up on you. Areas of your body that you were once proud to show off, you now keep covered up. Its time to find out why... and hit back!

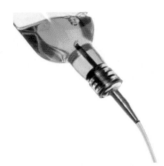

FAT... THE HARD FACTS

Fat contains no water or fibre yet it is dense in calories. You can consume large quantities of calories as fat without feeling full. For example, four tablespoons of vegetable oil contains nearly 700 calories. Yet four tablespoons of vegetable oil will not fill you up. You would need to consume four medium sized baked potatoes to take in 700 calories of carbohydrate. How full would you feel if you consumed four baked potatoes in one go?

700 calories of fat has to end up somewhere on your body. *How many thousands of calories in fat have you consumed over the years without realising where the fat will end up?*

Because fat contains no water or fibre, only energy, it weighs very little. Did you know that 700 calories in fat weighs less than three ounces? While four medium sized baked potatoes, containing the same number of calories, weigh one and a half pounds, mainly due to the additional water content of a potato.

SLOWLY & QUIETLY

Fat will build up on your hips, waist, thighs, buttocks and arms a little at a time. Fat works slowly and quietly. Try this. Go to where you keep your vegetable oil and pour around one pint of the vegetable oil into a clear container like a sandwich bag and then hold it up. That is one pound of fat. You are actually looking at more than 4,000 calories. That's right; one pound of fat contains more than 4,000 calories. If you were to cover it all over your body, you would soon realise that 4,000 calories in fat can be spread very thinly. Cunning or what?

Think carefully the next time you go to the salad bar, it's not the salad you have to watch, it's what goes on the salad that adds inches to your body. Fats love to hide in these areas camouflaged as healthy dressing, just waiting to ambush you. Even better, it's usually the potatoes or the bread that get the blame! If fat was a military force it would be attached to the SAS!

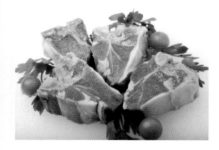

SATURATED FAT

Have you ever had a blocked sink or drain? It starts with a few things getting stuck in one area, usually a bend in the pipe. Over time, more and more debris becomes caught up until no water can get past. Consume too much saturated fat and you can create the same situation with far more serious consequences.

Saturated fat is the name given to fat that is solid at room temperature. We tend to see saturated fat as a white lump of lard, or the fat in red meat and in pies and pastries. But saturated fat comes in a variety of other different shapes, sizes and disguises.

Saturated fat is found in chocolates, biscuits, cakes, puddings and many of the sauces that make food come to life that you use every day.

THE KILLER

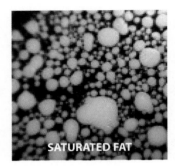

SATURATED FAT

Consuming too much saturated fat leads to an increase in your blood cholesterol levels of the bad type of cholesterol called low density lipoproteins (LDL). When too much LDL cholesterol is present in your blood it leads to a build up of fatty material in the blood vessels to your heart. Like the previous example of the blocked sink, these blood vessels can also become completely blocked causing a heart attack.

Remember that saturated fat comes in attractive snacks and tasty sauces.

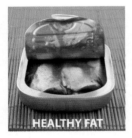

HEALTHY FAT

THE PARAMEDICS

The good news is that help is on hand in the form of the healthy fats. Consuming healthy fats also raises your blood cholesterol levels; they raise the levels of the good cholesterol called high density lipoproteins (HDL). HDLs are regarded as good because they carry excess cholesterol from your blood vessels back to the liver for disposal.

For good health it is important to change from consuming foods and snacks that are high in saturated fat to the healthy fats like nuts and avocado, especially the fish oils. In this way some healthy fats can be regarded as paramedics because they are associated with a decreased risk of coronary heart disease. Consuming oily fish a couple of times a week is recommended because of this.

However, to target a reduction in fat mass you also have to control both your saturated fat content and the amount of healthy fats you consume. In others words your total fat content.

A CHANGE IN FOCUS

Up to this point we have been discussing the energy in food in calories. However, when you look at nutritional information displayed on packets you will see that fat is not always shown in calories. It is shown in grams.

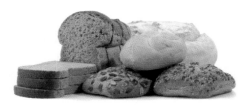

Nutritional Information per 100g	
Energy	433kJ/102kcal
Protein	1.2g
Carbohydrate	5.7g
Fat	8.3g

500g

This example shows the fat content as 8.3g per 100 grams of food.

TODAY WE USE GRAMS INSTEAD OF OUNCES.

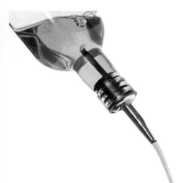

1 GRAM OF FAT
CONTAINS 9 CALORIES.

1 GRAM OF CARBOHYDRATE
CONTAINS 4 CALORIES.

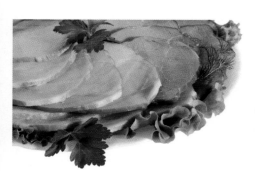

1 GRAM OF PROTEIN
CONTAINS 4 CALORIES.

BE WISE BEFORE YOU BUY

It will only take a few minutes or so of your time to help you uncover the myth behind some of the so-called low-fat foods. You will soon become aware of the hidden fat that is in your food.

Adopt the habit of quickly looking at *nutritional information* before you decide to buy. Go to where it shows the fat content and look at the number of grams of fat. By checking the fat content in this way, you could save yourself hours of physical slog.

THE BRITISH HEART FOUNDATION
So you want to lose weight... for good!

"Keeping the fat in your diet low is the best possible aid to weight loss and The Balance of Good Health is designed to do this "

"But remember fat is sometimes hidden in foods so it may not be obvious. Watch out! And always count the fat portions up to ensure you don't go over your daily or weekly limit."

FAT CONTENT PER 100 GRAMS OF FOOD
Sometimes when you look at the label displaying *Nutritional Information* it only shows this information per 100 grams of food. This means that you have to work out for yourself the total fat content per serving.

This example shows the fat content as 8.3g per 100 grams of food.

This is a five hundred gram jar of sauce. For every one hundred grams of sauce in this jar, you have 8.3 grams of fat. Therefore, the total fat content of the jar is 41.5 grams. (8.3g x 5). If this was being divided between two people, this would mean consuming around 20 grams of fat per person. You also have to take into consideration the fat content of the food that will be added to the sauce in the jar.

Nutritional Information per 100g	
Energy	433kJ/102kcal
Protein	1.2g
Carbohydrate	5.7g
Fat	8.3g

500g

The next example is another 500g jar of sauce. This jar of sauce has only 1.2g of fat per 100 grams of sauce. Then you multiply 1.2 by five to realise that there are only 6 grams of fat in this jar of sauce.

500g e

NUTRITIONAL DATA Per 100g (typical values)	
Energy	235kJ/55kcal
Protein	2.2g
Carbohydrate	8.8g
Fat	1.2g

THE TOTAL FAT CONTENT PER SERVING

This is much easier because the label shows you the total fat content based upon one serving.

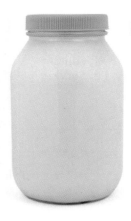

LOW-FAT SPREADS, DRESSINGS AND MAYONNAISE

The belief here is that because they are low in fat, you can consume larger portions than the original or full fat varieties. Although these do contain less fat than the original products, they are only low in fat if you use small amounts.

CHECK OUT THE HIDDEN FAT

*See where you are right now. How much hidden fat,
including the healthy fat, is in the foods you currently have
at home or buy from the shops?*

A FEW FACTS ABOUT FAT
- It will take the average woman, with a sedentary lifestyle, almost half the day to use up 30 grams of fat as energy.
- 4 tablespoons of Olive oil has 76 grams of fat.
- 1 medium sized avocado has around 20 grams of fat.
- 1 packet of peanuts (50g) has around 30 grams of fat.

Complete the table below you and give yourself an advantage right now. Look at the fat content of a few foods items you have at home today especially sauces, creams, spreads and frozen foods. Also look at the fat content of a few items before you buy and get ready for a real surprise!

FOOD ITEMS AT HOME	Fat Content Per 100g	Fat Content Per Serving
FOOD ITEMS SHOP BOUGHT	Fat Content **Per 100g**	Fat Content **Per Serving**

*Encourage your family to join in with you and help them also
appreciate the hidden fat content in foods.*

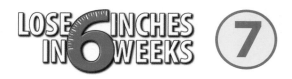

FAT CONTENT
OF
POPULAR FOODS

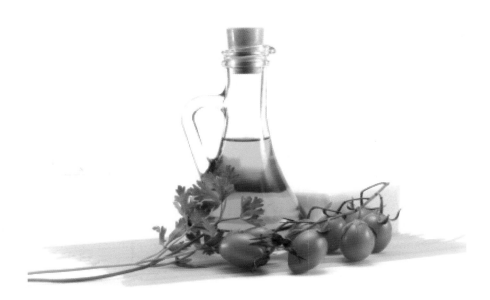

FOOD	Fat grams
BISCUITS 100g	
Assorted creams	25.7
Brandy snaps	20
Chocolate biscuits, fully coated	27.6
Cream biscuits	25
Custard creams	24
Digestive biscuits, plain	20.8
Crispbread, rye	2.5
Flapjacks	26.8
Hobnobs, milk chocolate biscuits	23.3
Jaffa cakes	10
Shortbread fingers	26.1
Water biscuits	12.8

BREADS	
Bagel, plain, average, 60g	0.5
Breadcrumbs, shop bought, 100g	2.1
Brown bread, average, 38g slice	0.8
Brown roll, crusty, 48g roll	1.3
Brown roll, soft, 48g roll	1.8
Chapatis, made with fat, 100g	12.2
Chapatis, made without fat, 100g	1
Croissant, 60g	12.5
Crumpet, wholemeal, 1 crumpet	0.4
Muffin, blueberry, 150g	13
Muffin, wholemeal, 67g	2

HARD FACTS

One gram of fat contains more than twice the number of calories than a combination of one gram of carbohydrate and one gram of protein.

Every gram of fat contains 9 calories.

To establish the number of calories from fat that there are in any of the food items, multiply each item grams of fat by 9 to convert to calories.

FOOD	Fat grams
CEREALS – BREAKFAST	
Bran flakes, 30g serving	0.6
Chocolate flavoured, rice pops, 30g serving	0.3
Cornflakes, 30g serving	0.2
Crunchy oat bran flakes, 30g serving	1.2
Fruit & fibre, 30g serving	1.4
Honey nut & cranberries, with 125ml of semi-skimmed milk, 30g serving	4.5
Muesli, Swiss style, 30g serving	1.8
Mulitgrain flakes, 30g serving	3
Porridge oats, made with 200ml semi-skimmed milk, 30g serving	4.5
Oats, porridge, rolled, 50g serving	4.5
Puffed wheat, 30g serving	0.4
Weetabix, 30g serving	0.9

FOOD	Fat grams
CEREALS – OTHER	
Flour, plain, white, 100g	1.3
Flour, wholemeal, 100g	2.2
Pasta, plain, all shapes, cooked, 265g serving	1.8
Rice, brown, boiled, 180g serving	2
Rice, fried, 190g serving	16
Rice, white, 190g serving	2.5
Spaghetti, white, boiled, 100g	0.7

FOOD	Fat grams
CHEESE 100g	
Brie	26.7
Cathedral City, light	21.4
Camembert	23.4
Cheddar	34
Cheddar, low fat	14.8
Cottage cheese, plain	3.9
Edam	25
Feta	19.8
Fromage frais	5.6
Full cream	18.8
Goats	14.8
Mozzarella	21.4
Parmesan	32.3
Soya cheese	26.4
Stilton	34.9

EGGS	
Small,1, 45g	4.9
Medium, 1, 55g	5.9
Large, 1, 60g	6.5
Large, fried, 1, 60g	8.3
Omelette, 2 eggs, 60g each	19.7
Poached, 1, 60g	6.5
Scrambled, 2 eggs, 60g each	27.1

FOOD	Fat grams
FATS, OILS & DRESSINGS	
Butter, 30g	24.5
Caesar dressing, 1 tbsp	7
Coco butter, 1 tbsp	20
Cod liver oil, 1 tbsp	20
Coleslaw, 1 tbsp	7
Coleslaw, light, 1 tbsp	3.5
French dressing, 100g	72.1
Garlic butter, 1 tbsp	16.5
Ghee, 100g	99.8
Lard 100g	99
Low-fat spread, 30g	12.1
Margarine, 30g	24.4
Mayonnaise, 1 tbsp	24.9
Mayonnaise, light, 1 tbsp	7
Mayonnaise, extra light, 1 tbsp	0.8
Olive oil, 30g	30
Olive oil, 1 tbsp	19
Potato salad, 1 tbsp	7
Salad cream, 100g	31
Thousand island dressing, 1 tbsp	7
Thousand island dressing, light, 1 tbsp	4

FISH & FISH PRODUCTS	
Cod in batter, fried, 100g	10.3
Cod, grilled, poached or baked, 100g	2
Eel, 100g	14.7
Fish fingers, grilled, per finger, average	2.5
Herring, grilled, 100g	13
Lemon sole, 100g	1.4

FOOD	Fat grams
FISH & FISH PRODUCTS CONTINUED	
Lumpfish, 100g	10
Mussels, 100g	2
Pilchards, canned in tomato sauce, 100g	5.4
Prawns, boiled, 100g	1.8
Salmon, 100g	12
Salmon, smoked, 100g	4.5
Sardines, canned in oil, drained, 100g	13.6
Sardines, fresh, 100g	11.6
Scampi, breaded and fried, 100g	17.5
Trout, rainbow, 100g	4.5
Tuna, canned, brine/water and drained, 100g	0.6
Tuna, canned in oil, drained, 100g	9

FOOD	Fat grams
FRUIT	
Apples, average, flesh and skin, 100g	0.1
Apricots, 100g	0.6
Avocado, average, flesh only, 100g	19.5
Bananas, no skin, 100g	0.3
Figs, dried, 100g	1.6
Grapefruit, flesh only, 100	0.1
Grapes, seedless, 100g	0.1
Kiwi fruit, whole, 100g	0.5
Fruit salad, canned in syrup, drained, 100g	0
Fruit salad, fresh, 100g	0.1
Mangoes, flesh only, 100g	0.2
Melon, honeydew, flesh only, 100g	0.1
Oranges, flesh only, 100g	0.1
Peaches, whole, 100g	0.1
Peaches, canned in syrup, 100g	0
Pears, whole, 100g	0.1
Pineapple, canned in juice, 100g	0
Plums, whole, average, 100g	0.1
Prunes, 100g	0.4
Strawberries, 100g	0.1

FOOD	Fat grams
MILK & YOGURTS	
Condensed milk, sweetened, 250ml	25.3
Evaporated milk, full fat, 250ml	23.5
Full fat milk, 250ml	9.8
Muller rice, low-fat, 200g	5
Semi-skimmed milk, 250ml	4
Skimmed milk, 250ml	0.3
Soya milk, 250ml	4.8
Soya milk, low-fat, 250ml	0
Yogurt, whole milk, plain, 200g	6
Yogurt, low-fat, fruit, 150g	1.1

MEAT & MEAT PRODUCTS	
Bacon, rashers, 2, 38g	26.6
Bacon, rashers, lean, 2, 32,	2.1
Beef, steak, grilled, 100g	6
Beef, mince, 100g	15.2
Beef burgers, frozen, fried, 100g	17.3
Beef, fillet steak, lean and trimmed, grilled, 100g	8.2
Black pudding, fried, 100g	21.9
Chicken breast, no skin, grilled, 100g	4
Chicken breast, with skin, grilled, 100g	9
Corned beef, canned, 100g	12.1
Ham, canned, 100g	5.1
Ham, slices, no added water, 1 slice, 25g	0.8
Lamb chop, lean grilled, 100g	12.3
Lamb chop, untrimmed, grilled, 100g	29
Lamb shank, lean, 100g	8.1
Pork crackling, 30g	18.7
Pork fillet, lean grilled, 100g	7.1
Pork loin chop, fat trimmed off, grilled, 100g	10.7
Pork loin, untrimmed, grilled, 100g	24.2
Pork pie, 180g	48.6

FOOD	Fat grams
MEAT & MEAT PRODUCTS CONTINUED	
Salami, 100g	45.2
Sausages, beef, grilled, 100g	17.3
Sausages, pork, grilled, 100g	24.6
Sausages, pork extra lean, 100g	13
Steak and kidney pie, 100g	21.2
Turkey, oven cooked, lean, 100g	2.7
Turkey, breast, no skin, 100g	1.4
Veal, loin chop, grilled, 100g	8.1
Veal, schnitzel, 100g	27
Veal, shank, lean, 100g	3

	Fat grams
NUTS	
Almonds, flesh only, 100g	55.8
Almonds, chocolate coated, 100g	44.6
Brazil, 100g	68.2
Cashew, 100g	45.7
Hazelnuts, 100g	63.4
Mixed nuts, 100g	54.1
Mixed nuts and raisins, 100g	34
Peanuts, roasted and salted, 100g	53
Pecan, 100g	70

	Fat grams
PASTA	
Egg, cooked, 100g	0.5
Plain, all shapes, cooked, 100g	0.2
Ravioli, cheese and spinach, cooked, 100g	6.2
Spinach, cooked, 100g	0.5
Ravioli, cheese & spinach, cooked, 100g	6
Tomato and herb fettuccine, 100g	0.7
Tortollini, cheese and spinach, cooked, 100g	6
Wholemeal, cooked, 100g	0.8

FOOD	Fat grams
PASTRY	
Filo, 1 sheet	0.3
Flaky, 100g	40.6
Puff, 100g	24.9
Shortcrust, 100g	32.3
Wholemeal, 100g	32.9

POTATO & POTATO PRODUCTS	
Baked potato, medium, 150g	0.3
Boiled, potatoes, 150g	0.5
Chips, homemade, fried in oil, 100g	6.7
Chips, oven baked, frozen, 100g	4.2
Mashed with skimmed milk, 100g	1
Roasted with skin, 100g	4.5

PUDDINGS & DESSERTS	
Apple pie, shop bought, 100g	15.5
Apple pie, low-fat, 100g	7
Apple strudel, 100g	11
Bread pudding, 100g	9.6
Cheesecake, frozen, 100g	10.6
Chocolate mousse, 100g	5.4
Chocolate sponge, 100g	26.3
Custard made with whole milk, 100g	4.5
Christmas pudding, 100g	9.7
Custard tart, 100g	14.5
Fruit crumble, 100g	6.9
Fruit pie, pastry top and bottom, 100g	13.3
Lemon meringue pie, 100g	14.4
Pavlova, shell mix, 100g	0
Pecan pie, 100g	18.2
Profiteroles, 100g	16.3
Rice pudding, canned, 100g	2.5
Soufflé, 100g	14.5
Tiramisu, 100g	20
Trifle, 100g	6.3

FOOD	Fat grams
SAUCES	
Bolognaise, 100g	11.1
Gravy, commercial, 100g	2.4
Hungarian goulash, 100g	3.4
Oyster, 1 tbsp	0
Pesto, 1 tbsp	0
Sweet & sour, 1 serving 115g	2.1
TOFU	
Fried, 100g	17.7
Burgers, 100g	9.5
Veggie burgers, 100g	9.5
VEGETABLES	
Aubergine, 100g	0.4
Beans, baked, canned in tomato sauce, 100g	0.6
Beans, red kidney, canned, drained, 100g	3
Beetroot, boiled, 100g	0.1
Brussels sprouts, 100g	1.4
Cabbage, raw, average, 100g	0.4
Carrots, old, boiled, 100g	0.4
Cauliflower, boiled, 100g	0.9
Courgette, raw, 100g	0.4
Cucumber, 100g	0.1
Lentils, red dried, 100g	1.1
Mushrooms, raw, 100g	0.5
Peas, frozen, 100g	1.5
Peppers, green, raw, 100g	0.3
Spinach, frozen, 100g	0.8
Sweet potato, 100g	0.3
Sweetcorn kernels, canned, 100g	1.2
Tofu, soya bean, 100g	4.2
Tomatoes, raw, 100g	0.3
Turnip, boiled, 100g	0.2
Watercress, 100g	1
YORKSHIRE PUDDING	
Small, 50g	4.9

FAST FOOD OUTLETS	Fat grams
BURGER KING	
Angus steak burger, 1, 276g	22
Bacon Cheeseburger, 1, 141g	19
Bagel, egg, cheese, sausage, 1, 203g	27
Chicken club, 1, 242g	32
Chicken fries, 6 pieces, 85g	15
Chicken whopper, 1, 272g	25
Veggie burger, 1, 272g	25
KENTUCKY FRIED CHICKEN	
Blazing twister s/w, 1, 246g	43
Chicken fillet burger, 1, 213g	19.2
Chicken pot pie, 1 serving, 243g	40
Crispy twister s/w, 1, 252g	38
Kentucky nuggets, 6 nuggets	18
Medium fries, 100g	14
McDONALD'S	
Bagel, ham, egg, cheese, 1, 218g	23
Big breakfast, 266g	46
Big Mac, 1, 219g	30
Cheeseburger, 1, 119g	12
Chicken McNuggets, 10 nuggets,	24
Medium fries, 100g	20

FAST FOOD OUTLETS	Fat grams
PIZZA HUT	
BBQ wings starter, per serving	22.2
Chicken and bacon salad, per serving	33.4
Lasagne, per serving	32.3
Muffin, mixed berry, 1	22.6
Pizza, farmhouse, medium pan, per serving	9.5
Pizza, Hawaiian, stuffed crust, per serving	14
Pizza, Margherita, medium pan, per serving	15

SUBWAY SANDWICHES	
6" Bourbon chicken, 1, 258g	5
6" Cheese steak, toasted, 1, 250g	10
6" Cheese and bacon ranch, 1, 296	25
6" Subway club, 1, 256g	6
6" Subway melt, 1, 254g	12
6" Tuna, 1, 250g	31

READY MEALS	Fat grams
BEEF LASAGNE	
Asda Beef Lasagne, frozen, 400g portion	14
Asda, Good for you lasagne, frozen, 400g portion	8.4
Chicago Town Deep Filled Lasagne Classic Beef, frozen, 250g portion	21.5
Co-op Italian Beef Lasagne, frozen, 340g portion	10
Co-op Italian Lasagne, fresh, 400g portion	21
Co-op Italian Healthy Living Beef Lasagne, fresh, 400g	8.4
Findus Beef Lasagne, frozen, 400g portion	13
Iceland Lasagne, frozen, 500g portion	18.9
M&S Beef Lasagne, fresh, 400 portion	38
M&S Count On Us…Beef Lasagne, frozen, 400g portion	7.6
Morrisons Beef Lasagne, frozen, 400g portion	29.6
Morrisons Eat Smart Diet…Lasagne, frozen, 400g	10.4
Sainsbury's Be Good To Yourself Lasagne, frozen, 450g portion	8
Sainsbury's Italian Lasagne, fresh, 376g portion	20.7
Sainsbury's Taste The Difference Beef Lasagne, fresh, 400g portion	32
Somerfield Healthy Choice Beef Lasagne, fresh, 430g	12
Somerfield Italian Beef Lasagne, fresh, 400g portion	22
Tesco Beef Lasagne, frozen, 450g portion	25.2
Tesco Healthy living Lasagne, frozen, 450g portion	10.3
Tesco Italian Lasagne, fresh, 400g portion	28
Waitrose Lasagne, fresh, 400g portion	22
Waitrose Perfectly Balanced Lasagne, fresh, 400g	8.8
Weight Watchers From Heinz Beef Lasagne, fresh, 400g portion	8.3
Weight Watchers Beef Lasagne, fresh, 400g portion	9.2

READY MEALS	Fat grams
CHICKEN TIKKA MASALA	
Asda Beef Indian Chicken Tikka Masala, fresh, 350g	21
Iceland Indian Takeaway Chicken Tikka Masala, frozen, 400g portion	28.3
M&S Tikka Masala Chicken, fresh, 175g portion	18.6
Morrisons Chicken Tikka Masala, fresh, 350g portion	36.5
Sainsbury's Chicken Tikka Masala, fresh, 200g portion	22.2
Somerfield Chicken Tikka Masala, fresh, 200g portion	27
Tesco Chicken Tikka Masala, fresh, 350g portion	26.1
Waitrose Chicken Tikka Makhani, fresh, 400g portion	30.4

CHEESE & TOMATO PIZZA	
Asda Fresh Cheese & Tomato Pizza, fresh, 190g	17.9
Asda Smart Price Cheese & Tomato Pizza, frozen, 121g portion	9.9
Chicago Town 5 Cheese Takeaway Original Pizza, frozen, 142.5g portion	15.1
Co-op Deep Pan Cheese & Tomato Pizza, frozen, 220g portion	18
Co-op Italian Stonebaked Margherita Pizza, frozen, 170g portion	11
Dr. Oetker Ristorante Pizza Mozzarella, frozen, 335g	48.3
Goodfella's Delicia Mozzarella, frozen, 131.5g	17.3
Iceland 12" Family Cheese Feast Pizza, frozen, 180g	19.9
Iceland Italian Stonebaked 5 Cheese Margherita, frozen, 205g portion	18.5
M&S Cheese & Tomato Pizza, fresh, 182.5g portion	15.1
M&S Cheese & Tomato Square Pizza, fresh, 138.8g	10.5
McCain Micro Pizza New & Improved Cheese & Tomato, frozen, 128g portion	16.5
McCain Pizza Fingers 10 Cheese 'N' Tomato (Grilled), frozen, 84g portion	6.7

READY MEALS	Fat grams
CHEESE & TOMATO PIZZA CONTINUED	
Morrisons Cheese & Tomato, fresh, 117g portion	9
Morrisons Margherita Pizza, fresh, 158g portion	12.7
Sainsbury's 3 Cheese & Tomato Pizzas, frozen, 91g	6.7
Sainsbury's Basics Cheese & Tomato Pizza, frozen, 121.5g portion	9.6
San Marco Snack Attack Pizza Fingers Cheese & Tomato, frozen, 135.5g portion	18.2
San Marco Snack Attack Pizza Minis Cheese & Tomato, frozen, 87g portion	8.4
Somerfield 3 Pizzas Cheese & Tomato, frozen, 82g	6.9
Somerfield Italian Style Thin & Crispy Margherita, frozen, 167.5g portion	21.2
Tesco 3 Tomato & Cheese Pizzas, frozen, 87g portion	6.9
Tesco Cheese Pizza, frozen, 197.5g portion	17.6
Waitrose Deep & Crispy Cheese & Tomato Pizza, fresh, 180g portion	17.1
Waitrose Thin & Crispy Cheese & Tomato Pizza, fresh, 152.5g portion	15.4
Weight Watchers Pizza Oval Cheese & Cherry Tomato, fresh, 93g portion	3

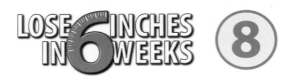
EASY
LOW-FAT MEALS

(Examples of meals with up to 10 grams of total fat)

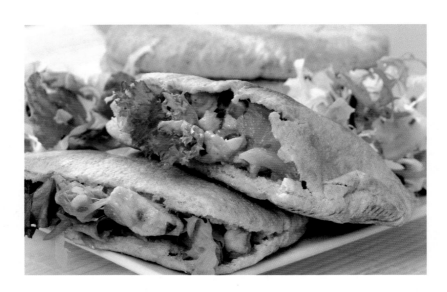

EASY LOW-FAT BREAKFASTS
Up to 10 grams of fat per meal (lose 0 points)

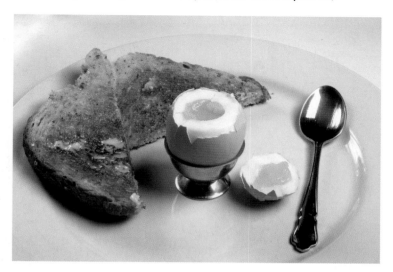

- Boiled or poached egg and 1-2 slices of brown toast with low-fat spread.

- Low-fat yoghurt with a handful of added raisins or sultanas.

- Banana milkshake made in a blender with one glass of semi-skimmed milk, one banana. A great energy booster!

- One or two slices of toast with low-fat spread and a little honey or jam.

FOOD FACT...
Using wholewheat bread gives you long-lasting energy. This applies to whole-grain breakfast cereals like Shredded Wheat too!

EASY LOW-FAT BREAKFASTS
Up to 10 grams of fat per meal (lose 0 points)

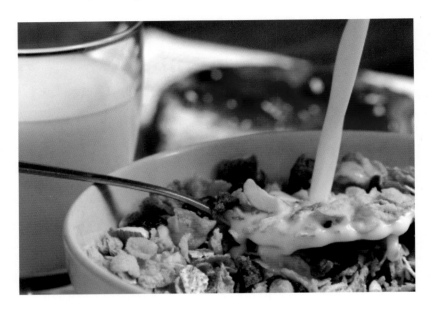

- Toasted pitta bread. Pop the pitta bread into a toaster. When toasted fill with a slice of low-fat cheese or a little honey or jam.

- Corn Flakes or Shredded Wheat with semi-skimmed milk or soya milk. Add some chopped banana or raisins for extra energy.

- Swiss style muesli with semi-skimmed milk. Add fresh fruit for extra fibre and vitamins to give you more energy.

EASY LOW-FAT BREAKFASTS
Up to 10 grams of fat per meal (lose 0 points)

- Unsweetened canned fresh fruit with low-fat yoghurt. Choose from pears, pineapple, peaches or mixed fruit.

- White or wholemeal muffin spread with a little low-fat spread, honey or jam.

- Fat-free fruit yoghurt and a glass of unsweetened fruit juice.

- Bagel with low-fat cream cheese.

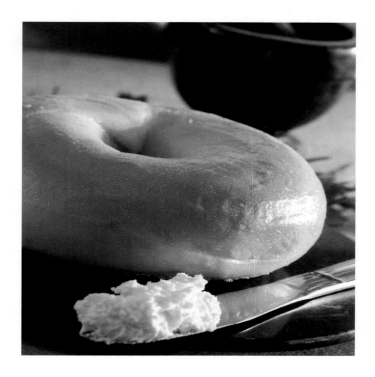

EASY LOW-FAT BREAKFASTS
Up to 10 grams of fat per meal (lose 0 points)

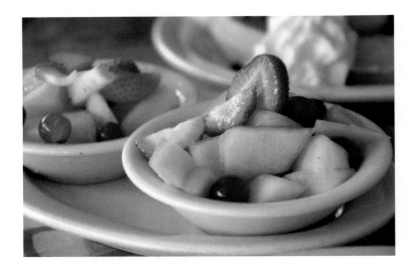

- Low-fat fruit yoghurt with added fresh chopped fruit and a teaspoon of sesame or sunflower seeds.

- 2 oatcakes spread with a little low-fat spread and honey or jam.

- Honey toastie. If you own a sandwich toaster why not make yourself a banana or honey-filled toastie using low-fat spread to coat the bread.

FOOD FACT...
Sesame seeds and sunflower seeds
contain healthy fats that help to keep your skin
and hair in good condition.

EASY LOW-FAT BREAKFASTS
Up to 10 grams of fat per meal (lose 0 points)

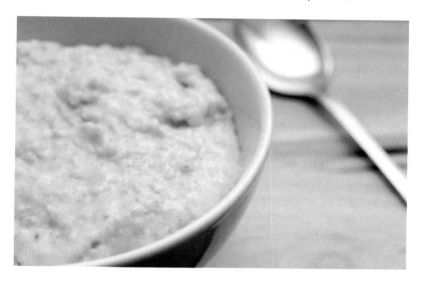

- Bowl of porridge oats with semi-skimmed or skimmed milk.

- Weetabix with semi-skimmed milk and a little sugar or honey.

- In a hurry? Why not grab a banana or a handful of raisins or sultanas.

FOOD FACT...
Bananas give you energy that lasts
because they contain starch; unlike sweets and
chocolate which only give you a quick burst of energy
and make you tired afterwards!

EASY LOW-FAT BREAKFASTS
Up to 10 grams of fat per meal (lose 0 points)

- Breakfast in a drink. Put 1 pot of low-fat yoghurt, 1 banana and some tinned peaches in a blender. Blend and drink.

- Soya or fat-free fruit yoghurt; add ½ teaspoon of sesame seeds with a glass of fresh orange juice.

- No cook quick porridge. Before going to bed, pour some oat-flakes into a breakfast bowl and cover with semi-skilled milk or soya milk. Add a little honey or some raisins and eat cold in the morning.

- Toasted English muffin with low-fat spread, honey, marmite or jam with a glass of milk.

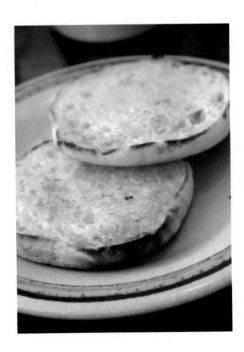

EASY LOW-FAT MEALS
Up to 10 grams of fat per meal (lose 0 points)

- Baked potato with tuna and sweetcorn mixed with 1 tablespoon of light mayonnaise. Serve with lettuce, tomato and cucumber.

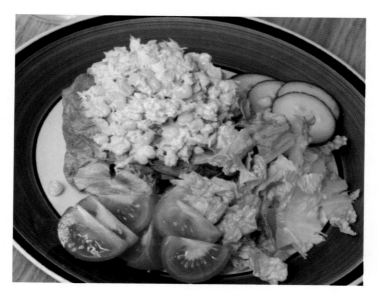

- Boiled rice with a savoury low-fat tomato sauce, tuna in brine or one chopped boiled egg. Add some diced vegetables such as carrots and peas.

- 2 Grilled fish cakes served with canned spaghetti in tomato sauce and a green salad.

FOOD FACT...
Brown (whole-grain) rice is better
than white because it releases its energy slowly –
this is why it's just great for losing weight!

EASY LOW-FAT MEALS
Up to 10 grams of fat per meal (lose 0 points)

- Super salad. Made with the likes of chopped tomatoes, sweetcorn, carrots, iceberg lettuce, cucumber, apple, courgettes, beetroot,   red kidney beans, sultanas, dates, etc. Add two tablespoonfuls of low-fat French dressing, or no-fat blue-cheese dressing. Serve with one small French bread stick or wholemeal roll, spread with a thin layer of low-fat spread.

- Prawn stir-fry. Fry prawns, peppers, courgettes and leeks together using fry light. Add a splash of soy sauce and a tablespoon of sweet chilli sauce. Serve with boiled rice mixed with peas, sweetcorn and peppers.

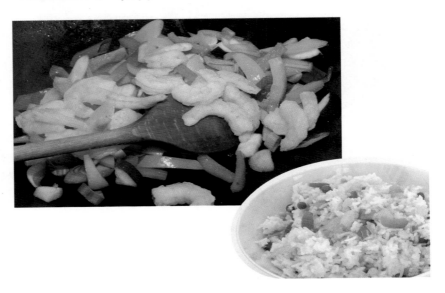

- Potato and carrot mash. Boil and mash the vegetables with one tablespoon of low-fat margarine; add a little salt and pepper. Serve with low-sugar baked beans and any of your favourite vegetables.

EASY LOW-FAT MEALS
Up to 10 grams of fat per meal (lose 0 points)

- Cod steak in a low-fat parsley sauce, with boiled or mashed potatoes, peas and carrots.

- Tuna and pasta bake. Cook some pasta, while the pasta is cooking fry an onion and a green pepper in a little fry light. Place the cooked pasta, fried onion, pepper with a tin of tuna and a tin of sweetcorn into an ovenproof dish. Add a jar of low-fat pasta sauce and mix together. Sprinkle a little low-fat grated cheese over the mix. Cook in the middle of oven for 50 mins at 200 degrees.

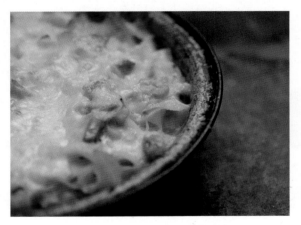

- Quorn-burger in a white or wholemeal roll spread with low-fat spread, iceberg lettuce and tomato ketchup; serve with low-fat oven chips.

- 3 fish fingers with new potatoes and steamed or lightly boiled cooked vegetables.

FOOD FACT...
Raw vegetables are full of vitamins
and enzymes that help to digest your meal.

EASY LOW-FAT MEALS
Up to 10 grams of fat per meal (lose 0 points)

- Cook wholemeal or white spaghetti; mix with low-fat pasta sauce and some cooked lean mince or turkey mince – serve with lightly cooked mixed vegetables. Drain any fat off the mince.

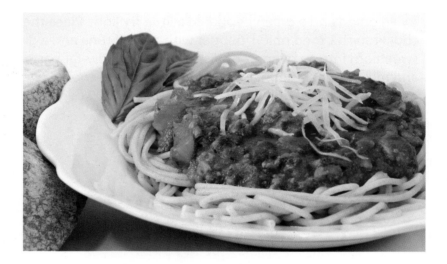

- Grilled or baked chicken with couscous and sweetcorn.

- 1 potato waffle with a pitta bread stuffed with tuna in brine and sweetcorn. Flavour with tomato ketchup or pickle.

- White or wholemeal pitta bread toasted and filled with a chopped boiled egg or a slice of low-fat cheese. Serve with a salad and flavour with tomato ketchup and pickle.

- Grilled parsnips, carrots, onions, garlic potatoes and courgettes. Wrap in foil, add some salt and pepper and bake in the oven. When cooked eat with a small French stick spread with a little low-fat spread. Add sauce or pickle.

EASY LOW-FAT MEALS
Up to 10 grams of fat per meal (lose 0 points)

- Pitta bread (wholewheat or white) filled with chicken. Serve with a salad.

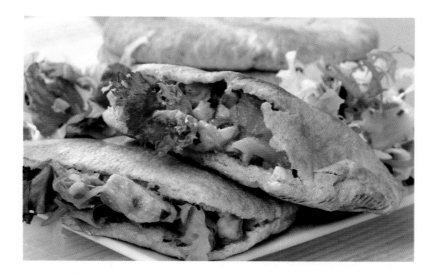

- Quorn banger and mash. Boil and mash the potatoes with salt, pepper and a little low-fat spread. Eat with 2 Quorn sausages and your favourite fresh vegetables.

- Grilled chicken breasts with pearl barley. Grill chicken on each side until golden and cooked through, then cut into slices. Fry the barley with some onion, chilli and green pepper in 1 teaspoon of olive oil. Serve the barley and vegetables topped with the chicken slices.

EASY LOW-FAT MEALS
Up to 10 grams of fat per meal (lose 0 points)

- Stuffed peppers. Cut open and clean out the seeds. Fill with boiled rice, baked beans, ham pieces and tomato sauce and bake in the oven.

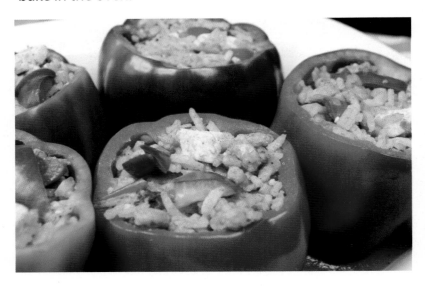

- Baked potato and pizza topping. Slice open the potato and add chopped mushrooms, green or red peppers and tomato sauce. Cook in microwave for 1 and ½ minutes. Grate some low-fat cheese as a topping.

- Potato wedges – cut 1 or 2 potatoes into wedge shapes; sprinkle with a little pepper and salt and coat with 1 teaspoon of olive oil; cook in the oven until crispy. Serve with your favourite vegetables.

EASY LOW-FAT MEALS
Up to 10 grams of fat per meal (lose 0 points)

- Grilled chicken with boiled or mashed potatoes and mixed diced vegetables in a low-fat sauce.

- Chicken and vegetable stir-fry. Slice chicken breasts into 1" chunks and stir-fry for 6-7 minutes or until golden using fry light. Transfer to a plate and keep warm. Cut the broccoli into florets, peel the carrots and cut into matchsticks. Blanch the broccoli in the boiling water for 2 minutes then drain well. Stir-fry the baby sweetcorn and carrots for 2 minutes using fry light. Stir in the broccoli and chicken then add a splash of soy sauce and a tablespoon of Hoi Sin sauce. Serve with wild rice.

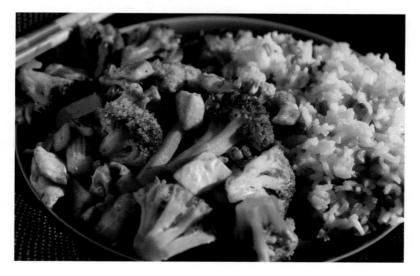

- Chicken casserole; place some lean chicken pieces in water along with your favourite vegetables in a casserole dish. Add a low-fat stock cube and cook in the oven. Eat with a piece of French stick or a slice of wholewheat bread spread with a thin layer of low-fat spread.

EASY LOW-FAT MEALS
Up to 10 grams of fat per meal (lose 0 points)

SOMETHING QUICK

- French stick filled with ham or chicken, a couple of low-fat cheese slices, iceberg lettuce and sliced tomato.

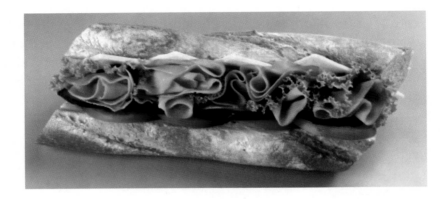

- Home-made curried beans on toast. Add some curry powder and sultanas to a can of baked beans, heat and eat on toast.

- ½ can of ratatouille with low-fat oven chips or baked potato; add a little low-fat grated cheese.

EASY LOW-FAT MEALS
Up to 10 grams of fat per meal (lose 0 points)

SOMETHING QUICK

Low-fat canned soups from Heinz, Baxters or Weight Watchers:

- Broccoli and watercress

- Garden pea and ham

- Spicy parsnip

  Eat with a white or whole-wheat roll or toast, spread with a little low-fat spread.

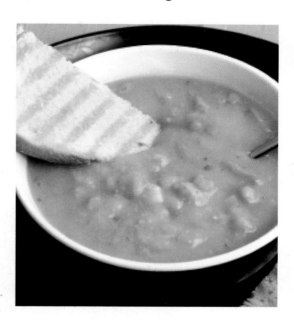

- Corn on the cob lightly cooked in water; coat with a little low-fat spread and eat with a salad.

- Canned pilchard fillets in tomato sauce on toast; serve with a green salad, and sweetcorn or low-sugar baked beans

EASY LOW-FAT MEALS
Up to 10 grams of fat per meal (lose 0 points)

SOMETHING QUICK

- Tuna sandwich with lettuce, cucumber and tomato. Add 1 teaspoon of low-fat mayonnaise. Remember to use tuna canned in brine, spring water but not oil.

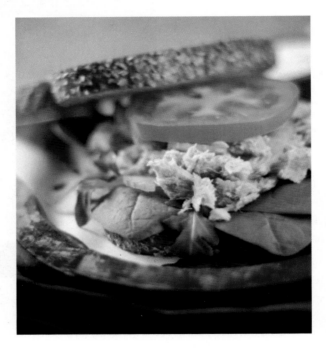

- 2 oatcakes with low-fat spreading cheese; serve with cherry tomatoes, carrot sticks and cucumber.

- Grate some carrots, add some raisins or sultanas; mix with some low-fat salad dressing or no-fat blue cheese.

EASY LOW-FAT MEALS
Up to 10 grams of fat per meal (lose 0 points)

SOMETHING QUICK

- Baked beans on toast with a little low-fat spread.

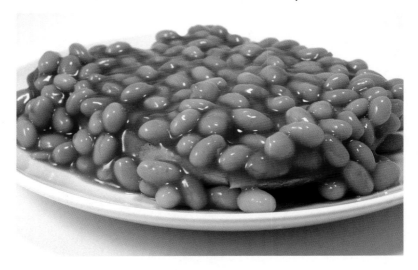

- Cheese toastie. Make a toastie with 1 slice of low-fat cheese; use a thin layer of low-fat spread to coat the bread; try adding some slices of tomato or onion.

- 2 rice-cakes spread with cottage cheese, marmite or 1 slice of low-fat cheese. Eat with a salad.

- 4 Ryvita crispbreads with a thin layer of low-fat humous or cottage cheese and cherry tomatoes.

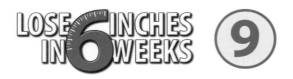

FAT BUSTING ACTIVITIES

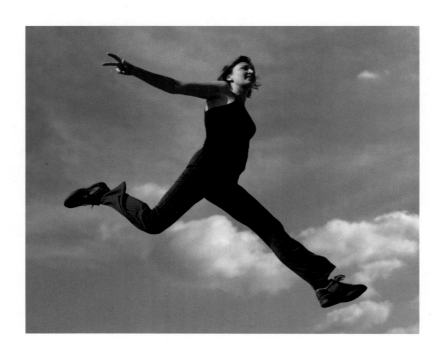

FAT BUSTING

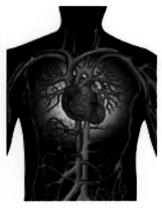

You may be surprised to know that your heart plays a major role in how much fat you lose from your body. When you involve activities that improve the strength of your heart, you also involve activities that help you to bust fat. Quite simply, fat busting and a healthy heart go hand in hand. This section will explain the link between developing a stronger heart and fat busting.

Your heart is a pump inside your body that sends blood carrying oxygen, food and nourishment to feed and nourish every living cell in your body. Used badly or ignored and your heart will weaken. Activities that you once found easy to do become much harder. Your energy levels drop and you become out of breath much quicker. Over time medical problems increase, you pile on the inches and feeling fit and healthy seems like a lifetime away.

Yet, with just a few easy activities, done regularly, your heart will become stronger and you will regain that healthy feeling. Whatever you do during the day affects your heart in one of two ways.

HEALTHY HEART

The first is related to improving the strength of your heart. Some activities will have a positive influence on improving the strength of your heart and some will not.

FAT BUSTING

The other aspect to consider is the amount of calories, especially fat, used as energy through these activities. The more calories from fat that you use as energy from your body the faster you become slimmer. The next few pages will discuss the effects of popular everyday activities from a view of both improving the strength of your heart and busting fat.

ACTIVITY - SITTING

The average office worker spends an average of six and a half hours *sitting* down at work; three hours *sitting*, eating, reading and watching TV and two hours commuting to work, usually *sitting*. Add on to that eight hours asleep and you begin to appreciate that we spend a lot of time saving energy and calories.

If you check your pulse and count the number of beats it makes in one minute when you are sitting down, you will usually have a pulse of between 60 to 80 beats per minute. The average is around 70 beats per minute. If you take into consideration that the maximum heart rate can go beyond 200 beats per minute, then a pulse of 70 beats per minute is low. It's low because your heart does not need to send much oxygen or food to your cells..

HEALTHY HEART

A pulse of around 70 beats per minute will result in no improvement in the strength or health of your heart. In fact, over time it can begin to get weaker. Instead of a pulse of 70 beats per minute when you are sitting down, it beats faster. A weak heart has to beat faster because it is not strong enough to pump out the same amount of oxygen with each beat.

FAT BUSTING

In addition, such a low pulse means that the demand from your muscle cells for food is also low. As your muscle cells are not expending much energy, then, you cannot be losing many calories, especially from fat. When you're sitting down or sleeping your body and uses fewer calories as energy. In this way your pulse is a good guide to the number of calories you are losing.

ACTIVITY - WALKING

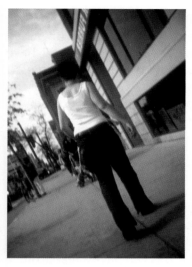

Walking is a very underrated and undervalued activity for improving good health and becoming slimmer. Occasionally, you may hear others say *"why walk and waste energy?"* The reality is that to become slimmer and healthier it's about wasting energy from all over your body.

HEALTHY HEART

As soon as you start moving around you bring into use some of the largest muscles in your body. These are the muscles of your buttocks, thighs and legs. Just normal walking will increase your pulse by around 10-20 beats every minute compared to sitting. As a result your heart is now pumping more oxygen, every minute, around your body. Although normal walking will not get you fit, it will get you active and that is a step in the right direction towards good health.

FAT BUSTING

Now here's the real surprise. By just increasing your heart rate by 10-20 beats per minute, you are now releasing twice as many calories than when you were sitting down. For every 10 minutes of normal walking, you are burning off twice as many calories than when you are sitting down.

ACTIVITY – BRISK WALKING

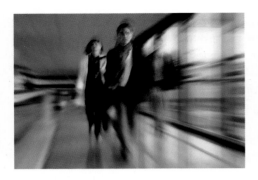

Brisk walking is a good way to improve your health and is such a positive aid to slimming. In the 35 years I have been involved with health & fitness I would rate brisk walking as one of the best lifestyle activities that you can do outside the gym environment to help you become slimmer.

HEALTHY HEART

Normal walking will increase your pulse by around 10-20 beats every minute compared to sitting. Brisk walking will raise your pulse even further, by as much as 20-30 beats per minute. This means that your heart is now pumping a great deal more oxygen every minute around your body. This can have a real positive effect on improving both the strength and health of your heart.

FAT BUSTING

Remember that as soon as you start moving around you bring into use some of the largest muscles in your body. The muscles of your buttocks, thighs and legs have to use many more calories from fat through brisk walking than when you are sitting down. For every 10 minutes of brisk walking you do, you are burning up nearly three times more calories from fat than when you are sitting down.

STEP UP YOUR DAILY ACTIVITY LEVELS

Look to move that little bit quicker every day, especially when walking around. Your heart will benefit and you will use more calories from fat as a result.

DEVELOP A FAT BUSTING LIFESTYLE

- Look for a parking space that means you have to walk further.

- Plan to give yourself an extra 10 minutes in the morning and afternoon as part of your walking slimming programme.

- Go for a walk at lunchtime, even if it is just around the shops. Walking will release twice as many calories as sitting down and surfing the net.

- Be aware of the length of time you spend sitting down. When possible, take regular activity breaks.

- If your waste paper basket is by your desk, move it. Try putting it on the other side of your desk. You have to get up each time you want to put something in it. It's a pain to start with but stick with it.

- If you have a short report or something similar to read, then stand up and walk around as your read. The extra oxygen generated from moving around, passes through your brain, and will help with your concentration.

- When you have to move a few things from one place to the next, only take one or two at a time.

- If you have young children, include some activity time with them. Playing is such a great way to encourage children to be active and to entice them away from the TV.

- Walking up and down stairs is exercise and a great way to help tone up your legs, thighs and buttocks through your lifestyle. Using the stairs immediately boosts the amount of calories your body releases as energy. Start to see your stairs in your house as part of your home gym equipment and let your family into this secret.

FORMAL EXERCISES

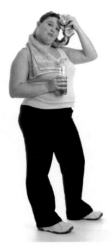

These include activities like cycling, swimming, jogging, games and sports, gym workouts, exercise classes and power walking.

As a very general guideline the exercises listed above can usually raise your pulse rate higher than that of walking and brisk walking.

HEALTHY HEART

Some of the exercises listed above have the advantage of doing more than improve general health. They can also strengthen your muscles, joints and bones. In addition, they will help to keep you supple and of course they raise your fitness levels. The key here is to walk before you run. Keep your pulse rate at a comfortable level for you. Let your body get used to walking first. Then gently introduce brisk walking before you think about moving onto the higher intensity activities.

This is one of the advantages of joining a gym, as a fitness professional can put together the right programme for your current level of fitness.

FAT BUSTING

All of the activities shown above use the large muscle groups of your buttocks, thighs and legs. Some of these have the benefits of introducing other areas like your arms, back and tummy. Collectively, they can release three to four times more calories from fat than sitting down. As a result you can see and feel the difference much sooner.

OTHER BENEFITS

Exercise also offers a relief from mild depression. You produce a greater amount of chemicals in your body that make you feel good about yourself and exercise will help you see results much faster. The important aspect with exercise is that you enjoy what you are doing. So look to try a wide range of formal activities until you find the one you enjoy the most.

IF YOU ARE A GYM USER

Even if you do regular physical exercise, be aware of your activity levels outside of the gym environment. It is all those little movements you make, some that take just 30 seconds that will all count in the end. There are 168 hours in a week, even if you workout three times a week, it's what you're doing for the other 165 hours that will help to make a difference.

FIDGET AWAY THE FAT

In current research scientists at the Mayo Clinic in Rochester, Minnesota found out that lean people spend more than 2½ hours longer each day standing and moving around than those who were overweight.

The scientists claim that lean people can burn off an extra 350 calories a day through this behaviour – equivalent to an intensive 45 minutes workout.

Dr James Levine, who led the US study said: 'Our study shows that the calories that people burn in their everyday activities are far, far more important in weight loss than we previously imagined.'

The scientists used a system of electronic sensors which were attached to volunteers to monitor their movements 24 hours a day for ten days.

Make activity an integral part of your lifestyle outside the gym environment. If you combine an active lifestyle with the benefits of any gym or exercise class then you are onto a real winner.

GOOD POSTURE COUNTS

Have you ever watched any of those costume dramas where the lady and the gentleman are always sitting bolt upright? Give it a try and see how long you last before your muscles start to weaken.

One of the best ways to condition specific muscles of your body is through being aware of general good posture. It's also the most natural way. Give this a bash. Go and stand in front of a mirror sideways on. Then pull your tummy in, now pull it in even more. How does it feel, can you feel the muscles of your tummy and back working? You're doing a new type of exercise that's called *Upright Isometric Abdominal Conditioning.*

Isometric conditioning is a way to develop muscle conditioning without much movement. When you do tummy curls you work your tummy muscles by means of movement, you curl your tummy up and down. The technical name for this type of conditioning work is called isotonic conditioning. Yet both isotonic and isometric exercises will condition your tummy.

The advantage of *Upright Isometric Abdominal Conditioning* is that you can do this any time; when you're walking, sitting watching TV or even driving your car. Pull your tummy in, hold it for two or three seconds, and then release it again. Keep repeating this during the day.

When you are in the home, at work or even shopping, you can carry out this exercise. It's an easy way to naturally condition some of the muscles of your upper body. Even if you are a regular gym user, working on good posture outside the gym will bring you rewards.

IT'S ALL IN THE BAG

Have you ever been surprised at how much air you can blow into a balloon and then watch the balloon release the air and go back to the same size again?

Your tummy acts a bit like a balloon. It's a bag hanging inside your body. When it's full of food you can easily think that you have got fatter. Your clothes feel tighter, you feel full and usually feeling full is often accompanied by feeling fat. When it's empty it gives you the impression that your tummy is flat.

You can prove this yourself. Check your tummy in the mirror before your sit down for your evening meal and then check it again just afterwards and you will see how much it has expanded. This is because of the food waiting in your tummy to be broken down and sent into your body. High fibre foods take up additional space in your tummy through the fibre, which increases the size of your tummy after any meal.

Once the food has been broken down, the energy (calories) from food will be sent into your body. Any fibre will also leave your tummy to be passed out of your body.

Even if you have a flat tummy after a high-fibre meal, your tummy will look bigger. Do not be fooled by the ever expanding and decreasing size of your tummy. It's just the bag inside you. It's when food leaves your tummy and those calories hit your blood stream that the damage is done to increase the size of your fat mass.

You can sometimes become so focussed on what is happening to your ever-changing waistline, that you do not notice what is happening to the other areas of your body. Areas like the little lumps on your back, your love handles and the fat on the back of your arms. All of these can be diminishing so remember to look at these changes just as much as you look at your tummy.

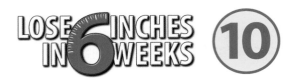

CARBOHYDRATE
UNCOVERED

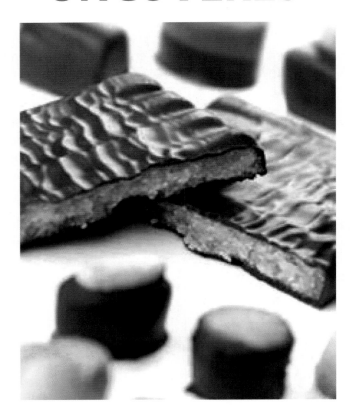

THE ENERGY PROVIDER

In the summer of 1989 I headed a team of full and part time fitness professionals with the responsibility of setting up and running a brand new local authority gym complex, it was called a fitness studio in those days. Part of my responsibilities was to set up and manage the regular induction courses. Induction courses became the format for introducing new members to the correct use of the various machines in the gym and their individual exercise programmes. Nearly 3,000 new members were taken through these induction courses under my management.

As with any gym, there were incidents and accidents that occurred. Some you would be really surprised at. One person slipped a disc in his back when altering the seat height on the chest press. Another dislocated his shoulder reaching up to grab the bar on the lateral pull down. Yet, the most common incidents that I can recall related to people feeling faint just after starting their exercise programme or induction course. On one particular Sunday alone, three new members felt very faint on three consecutive induction courses. Two of these were diabetic and needed sugar fast to stop them from going into hypo.

Unlike fat, where we can easily store up to 90,000 calories in our fat mass, we only hold a very limited amount of sugar.

SUGAR

Sugar is the common name given to the type of sugar used as energy by your body. The proper name is glucose. Because blood glucose is commonly called blood sugar, this can be confused with refined sugar but it is very different. Regularly consuming refined sugar can lead to serious health issues like type 2 diabetes and dental health problems.

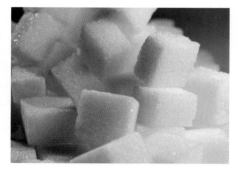

GLUCOSE

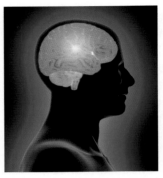

Glucose on the other hand is essential in combining with fat to supply your muscles with energy.

Crucially, glucose also nourishes the cells of the brain and the nervous system. This is taken from the glucose circulating in your blood stream. Around 500 calories a day of glucose is used by your brain and nervous system. Even when you are asleep glucose from your blood stream has to continue to nourish the cells of your brain and nervous system. That is why a light evening snack can help you to sleep better through the night.

When your blood glucose levels drop too low, you not only feel hungry, but also irritable. Your concentration is reduced and you move slower, even in the gym. Low blood glucose levels can also lead you to making the worst possible choices for snacks. It is low blood glucose that can drive you to eating too much in one go, or even bingeing.

STORED ENERGY

The average person's store of fat is more than 50 times greater than their store of glucose. An overweight person's store of fat can be 100 times greater than their store of glucose. Which energy source are they going to run out of first, fat or glucose?

When you exercise, or you are physically active you increase both the amount of fat and glucose that you use as energy. You can see how easy it is to take your blood glucose levels to the edge, especially if you skip breakfast and then go to the gym in the morning. So where do you get glucose from?

CARBOHYDRATE

Glucose comes from the metabolism (from the Greek word for change) of carbohydrate. Foods that contain carbohydrate are absorbed into your intestines, where the carbohydrate part is broken down into glucose.

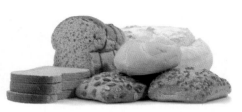

Glucose is then sent into your body and is changed again into energy that can be used by your muscles and to nourish the cells of your brain and nervous system. A limited amount of glucose is also stored in your muscles and liver as your glucose reserve. The bad news is that glucose can also be changed into fat.

It is when too much glucose is broken down from carbohydrate, especially at one time, that this increases the risk of glucose being changed into fat. That's why, by controlling the total amount of the carbohydrate you consume, you also control the amount of glucose you release.

In reality, there are really only three possible outcomes regarding carbohydrate and glucose and these are:

1. **A High Carbohydrate Intake**
   You consume too much carbohydrate and thus you release too much glucose into your blood stream.

2. **A Low Carbohydrate Intake**
   You do not consume enough carbohydrate and therefore your blood glucose levels remain low.

3. **A Balanced Carbohydrate Intake**
   You consume the right amount of carbohydrate and at the right times. This creates the ideal situation.

A HIGH CARBOHYDRATE INTAKE

High carbohydrate diets or food plans just do not make any sense as the additional carbohydrate not used as energy, or stored in the liver, will be changed into fat.

The flow chart below shows the eventual outcome of consuming too much carbohydrate. Although both the muscles and the cells of the brain and nervous system are receiving glucose, it's what happens to the additional glucose that causes the problem.

HIGH CARB INTAKE

A lot of glucose released and sent into the body more than the brain and muscles can use as energy.

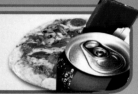

1. Brain Cells

Glucose from the blood stream provides the brain and nervous system with enough energy to maintain good concentration.

2. Muscle Cells

Glucose also supplies the muscles with energy for movement.

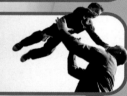

3. Liver Cells

Glucose not used by the brain and muscles is stored in the liver for use later.

4. Glucose to Fat

Any excess glucose is converted into fat in the liver and then sent into the fat cells.

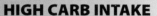

FOODS CONTAINING CARBOHYDRATE

One of the questions I ask at the group workshops that I run is to name some foods that contain carbohydrate. Immediately the usual suspects are highlighted such as bread/rolls, potatoes, cereal, rice and pasta.

There have been very few occasions when someone responds to my question and says chocolates, biscuits, cakes, puddings, pizzas, curries and soft sugary drinks.

In fact, these all contain carbohydrate in varying amounts. The difference is that some of the foods in the latter group contain refined sugar, like the chocolates, biscuits, cakes and puddings. This is the worst type of carbohydrate.

These foods taste nice because of the sugar content. The other issue is that many of the foods shown in the latter group are very high in carbohydrate and also contain fat. This increases the total calorie content of the foods to high calorie.

TIME TO MOVE ON
With so many foods, snacks and drinks containing carbohydrate you can understand just how easy it is to consume too much carbohydrate without realising this.

It's time we moved on from just looking at bread, cereals, potatoes, rice and pasta as carbohydrate foods and appreciate the high carbohydrate value of many other foods and snacks. I believe that it is also time we moved on from just showing the sugar content and show the total carbohydrate content.

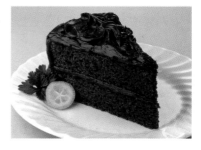

A LOW CARBOHYDRATE INTAKE

One thing is for sure, that on a low carbohydrate intake, no glucose will be converted into fat. There are other unhealthy side effects that you must consider. Energy levels drop through a lack of glucose in the muscles. Plus poor concentration through a drop in the circulating blood glucose and possible muscle wastage.

LOW CARB INTAKE
Not enough glucose released and sent into the body.

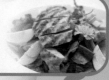

1. Brain Cells
Poor concentration due to lack of glucose.

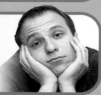

2. Muscle Cells
A general feeling of sluggishness leads to low activity levels.

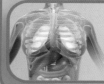

3. Liver Cells
Glucose stored in the liver is used as energy by the brain and muscles. Live stores of glucose become depleted. Some protein has now to be converted into glucose to cover the shortfall.

No short term nutritional deficiency (except lack of water) is more immediately apparent than a drop in blood sugar. When the level of glucose in our blood falls out of the normal range, we not only feel hungry but irritable, sluggish and depressed as well. "While all the body cells consume some glucose, two thirds of the glucose we need go to nourish the cells of the brain and nervous system. These cells depend upon glucose almost exclusively. Without it, they die.

PAUL SALTMAN (Nutritional Scientist) Professor of Biology at UCSD

THE ATTRACTION OF THE LOW CARBOHYDRATE DIETS

The attraction of a low carbohydrate diet is that you get immediate weight loss from the reduction of essential glucose and water lost from your muscles and liver but you may not be losing any fat!

For every one pound of stored glucose you lose from your body you also lose almost 2½ times that weight again in water (a total of 3½ pounds). Yet losing stored glucose and water is not the same as losing stored fat.

That is why you can see quick results on the scales but not on your fat mass through low-carbohydrate diets. The weight has been lost from inside your body mass, initially from water and glucose but then it gets worse as you continue with a low-carb diet.

MUSCLE WASTAGE AND AN INCREASE IN CELLULITE

Have you every seen anyone who has had a broken leg put into a plaster cast? The muscle in the leg very quickly wastes away, becomes smaller, thinner, and weaker and loses its shape. Now imagine the leg being surrounded by fat. All you would see from the outside is a thinner leg.

In the absence of carbohydrate, your body has to find glucose from somewhere. The answer is to convert protein into glucose. Some of the protein that should be used to keep lean body mass healthy is converted into glucose. The result is that your body mass begins to waste away just like the example of the broken leg and cellulite can increase between your depleted lean mass and fat mass.

It is this fast weight loss that gets you hooked at the start and why the most common type of fad diet has been a low carbohydrate diet, because of this immediate weight loss from glucose and water. The only thing that changes with a low-carbohydrate diet is the name. The messages are the same though, cut out bread, potatoes and rice and you can lose five pounds in the first few days. These are foods that come from mother earth that have nourished millions of people for thousands of year. Low-carb diets will keep coming, what will the next one be called?

A BALANCED CARBOHYDRATE INTAKE

This is the best way to get through each day. You replace the glucose used as energy in your muscles and liver, which allows you to be more active later. Continually topping up the glucose levels in your blood stream is good for your concentration and alertness. With no additional glucose being consumed, then no glucose will be converted into fat. This creates a win – win situation for you every day

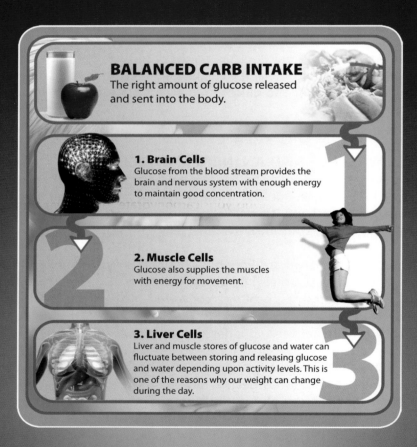

BALANCED CARB INTAKE
The right amount of glucose released and sent into the body.

1. Brain Cells
Glucose from the blood stream provides the brain and nervous system with enough energy to maintain good concentration.

2. Muscle Cells
Glucose also supplies the muscles with energy for movement.

3. Liver Cells
Liver and muscle stores of glucose and water can fluctuate between storing and releasing glucose and water depending upon activity levels. This is one of the reasons why our weight can change during the day.

HOW MUCH CARBOHYDRATE SHOULD YOU CONSUME?

There are clear guidelines for carbohydrate intake. These guidelines are also displayed as part of nutritional information.

GUIDELINE DAILY AMOUNTS

	Women	Men	Children (5-10 years)
Carbohydrate	**230g**	**300g**	**220g**
of which **sugar**	90g	120g	85g

The reality is that we are all different and have varying lifestyles. If you are small, and leading a sedentary lifestyle then these guidelines could be too high. Alternatively, if you're tall and very active, and exercise, then these guidelines could be too low.

What is known is that your total store of glucose is very limited and needs to be regularly topped up. By spreading your carbohydrate intake over three meals and two to three snacks, instead of just three meals, you actually consume less carbohydrate at one time. This reduces the possibility of too much glucose being sent into your body at one time.

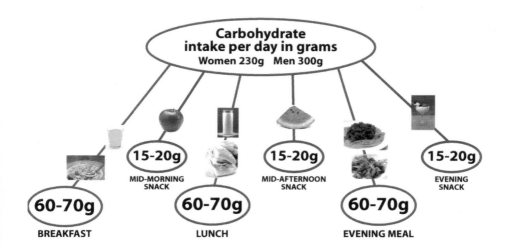

Carbohydrate intake per day in grams
Women 230g   Men 300g

15-20g — MID-MORNING SNACK
15-20g — MID-AFTERNOON SNACK
15-20g — EVENING SNACK
60-70g — BREAKFAST
60-70g — LUNCH
60-70g — EVENING MEAL

EMOTIONAL SIGNALS

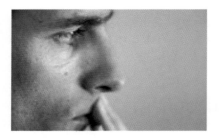

How good are you at listening to the signals your body sends you? Your body communicates to you through a series of emotional signals. When your blood glucose levels begin to drop your brain starts sending messages to prod you to top up your blood glucose levels.

The initial signal starts with you feeling a bit peckish. If you ignore this one, your body sends out a stronger signal to eat. If you also ignore this, then the situation will only deteriorate.

The lack of glucose in your blood stream means that there is not enough energy currently available for your brain, so it cannot work efficiently. Even though your muscles can be full of energy, your brain slows the rest of your body down to conserve blood glucose. Other symptoms include:

- Feeling really hungry and you need to eat something fast.
- You can become irritable and sometimes hands start to tremble.
- Feeling lethargic and tired. You move slower to conserve energy.
- Encourages bingeing on high sugar/high fat snacks with sugar levels shooting up into the high-sugar category because too much carbohydrate has been consumed.
- Even though your glucose levels are high they can quickly be lowered through the release of insulin.
- Risk of some glucose being changed into fat.
- Regularly increasing your blood glucose levels high can lead to type 2 diabetes.

SUGAR LEVELS	BLOOD SUGAR LEVELS
High-Sugar	
Time to Eat	
Very-low Sugar	

BREAK THE FAST

Skipping meals, especially breakfast encourages this situation later in the morning. Breakfast is the meal that is easiest to miss as you may not feel hungry first thing in the morning. Overnight your body has basically been fasting. Breakfast means breaking the fast. By topping up your blood glucose levels soon after you wake up you are breaking the fast and setting your body up to burn energy faster.

BRITISH NUTRITION FOUNDATION

"Overnight while you have been asleep, your metabolism slows down, so eating soon after you wake up helps to boost your metabolism and gets the body going again."

"That's not all; research has shown that skipping the first meal of the day may lead to an unhealthy pattern of snacking on high-fat foods throughout the morning."

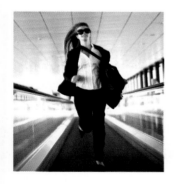

By planning to start the day with breakfast, you are giving your body a 'kick-start' to the day. Breakfast does not have to be a cooked meal, a simple bowl of cereal will do. If you get up late and are in a rush, try a glass of fruit juice and take a breakfast cereal bar with you to eat on the way. The key is to put some energy into your body to top up your blood glucose levels and get your mind and body active and into gear at the start of the day.

If you have been continually skipping breakfast and you never feel hungry in the morning, then when you start having breakfast, you will notice a surprising change. After about four days you will receive a different message, one that says 'I feel hungry and need to eat something.'

EAT EVERY THREE TO FOUR HOURS

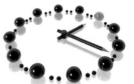

By listening to the signals that your body sends out, and acting on them before your glucose levels drop too low, you can make better choices and will not feel compelled to eat so much carbohydrate in one go.

By spreading your carbohydrate intake across the whole day and eating every three to four hours, you consume smaller amounts of carbohydrate. The advantages are:

- Your concentration is good.

- Your energy levels are maintained.

- This will prevent your blood glucose levels rising too high.

- Your blood sugar levels become more stable, which prevents you craving high sugar snacks.

In some cases by controlling your total fat intake, you will also be controlling your carbohydrate intake. However, there will be times when you will need to control your carbohydrate intake as well. By replacing some carbohydrate with protein you end up consuming the same amount of calories.

Protein when mixed in a meal with carbohydrate actually slows down the rate at which your body digests carbohydrate into glucose. Simple things such as having a smaller baked potato or portion of rice or pasta and adding a filling like tuna or chicken are examples of how to do this.

SUGAR LEVELS	BLOOD SUGAR LEVELS
High-Sugar	
Time to Eat	
Very-low Sugar	

FILL UP ON GOODNESS

It is also important that you look to choose the best types of carbohydrate for your meals, snacks and drinks. Here are a few tips to help you to do this.

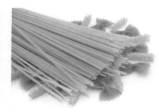

Include starchy carbs with each meal.

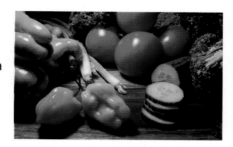

Add fresh or frozen vegetables or salad with as many meals as possible.

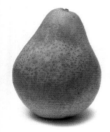

Fresh fruit is your ideal mid-morning and mid-afternoon snack.

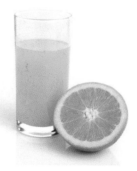

Adopt the habit of enjoying a glass of fresh fruit juice as part of your breakfast. This counts as part of your five a day for fruit and vegetables. It will also give you an additional 20-25 grams of carbohydrate in the morning.

FRUIT & VEGETABLES...
WHAT'S A PORTION?

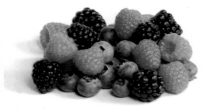

1 medium fruit: apples, bananas, pears, nectarines, slice of melon and peaches.

2 small fruits: plums, satsumas, kiwi fruits and apricots.

1 cupful of berry type fruit: cherries, raspberries, grapes, and strawberries.

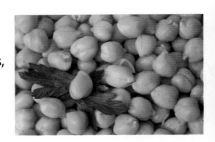

Half a cupful of pulses: chickpeas, baked beans, kidney beans and lentils.

1 glass of fruit juice.

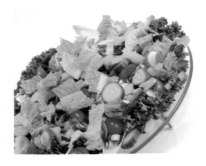

1 dessert bowlful of mixed salad vegetables, lettuce and salad leaves.

2 tablespoons of cooked vegetables: carrots, green beans, broccoli and cauliflower.

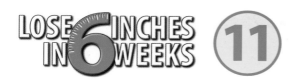

CARBOHYDRATE CONTENT OF POPULAR FOODS

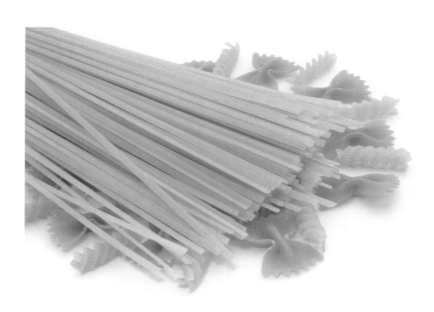

FOOD	Carbs grams
BISCUITS 100g	
Assorted creams	68.5
Brandy snaps	64
Chocolate biscuits, fully coated	67.6
Cream biscuits	64
Custard creams	64
Digestive biscuits, plain	67.9
Crispbread, rye	70
Flapjacks	60.4
Hobnobs, milk chocolate biscuits	60.7
Jaffa cakes	68.8
Shortbread fingers	63.9
Water biscuits	65.3

BREADS	
BREADS	
Bagel, plain, average, 60g	29
Breadcrumbs, shop bought, 100g	78.5
Brown bread, average, 38g slice	16.8
Brown roll, crusty, 48g roll	24.2
Brown roll, soft, 48g roll	24.9
Chapatis, made with fat, 100g	48.3
Chapatis, made without fat, 100g	43.7
Croissant, 60g	23
Crumpet, wholemeal, 1 crumpet	17
Muffin, blueberry, 150g	56
Muffin, wholemeal, 67g	27

HARD FACTS

Every gram of carbohydrate contains only 4 calories.
To establish the number of calories from carbohydrate
that there are in any of the food items,
multiply each item grams of carbs by 4 to convert to calories.

FOOD	Carbs grams
CEREALS – BREAKFAST	
Bran flakes, 30g serving	20.8
Chocolate flavoured, rice pops, 30g serving	28.3
Cornflakes, 30g serving	25.8
Crunchy oat bran flakes, 30g serving	22.2
Fruit & fibre, 30g serving	21.6
Honey nut & cranberries, with 125ml of semi-skimmed milk, 30g serving	27
Muesli, Swiss style, 30g serving	22.7
Mulitgrain flakes, 30g serving	21.5
Porridge oats, made with 200ml semi-skimmed milk, 30g serving	24.1
Oats, porridge, rolled, 50g serving	40.2
Oat cereal, with raisins, almonds and honey, 50g serving with 125ml semi-skimmed milk	50.1
Puffed wheat, 30g serving	20.2
Weetabix, 30g serving	22.7

CEREALS – OTHER	
Flour, plain, white, 100g	77.7
Flour, wholemeal, 100g	63.9
Pasta, plain, all shapes, cooked, 265g serving	24.7
Rice, brown, boiled, 180g serving	57.8
Rice, fried, 190g serving	56
Rice, white, 190g serving	58.7
Spaghetti, white, boiled, 100g	22.2

FOOD	Carbs grams
CHEESE	
Brie, 30g	0
Cathedral City, light, 30g	0
Camembert, 30g	0
Cheddar, 30g	0
Cheddar, low fat, 30g	0
Cottage cheese, plain, 30g	0.6
Edam, 30g	0
Feta, 30g	0
Fromage frais, 30g	4.1
Full cream, 30g	1.2
Goats, 30g	0
Mozzarella, 30g	0
Parmesan, 30g	0
Ricotta, 30,	0
Soya cheese, 30g	0
Stilton, 30g	0

EGGS	
Small,1, 45g	0
Medium, 1, 55g	0
Large, 1, 60g	0
Large, fried, 1, 60g	0
Omelette, 2 eggs, 60g each	0
Poached, 1, 60g	0
Scrambled, 2 eggs, 60g each	0.7

FOOD	Carbs grams
FATS, OILS & DRESSINGS	
Butter, 30g	0
Caesar dressing, 1 tbsp	3
Coco butter, 1 tbsp	0
Cod liver oil, 1 tbsp	0
Coleslaw, 1 tbsp	7
Coleslaw, light, 1 tbsp	5
French dressing, 1 tbsp	5.5
French dressing, low-fat, 1 tbsp	3.5
Garlic butter, 1 tbsp	0
Ghee, 1 tbsp	0
Lard	0
Low-fat spread, 30g	0.1
Margarine, 30g	0.3
Mayonnaise, 1 tbsp	0.6
Olive oil, 30g	0
Olive oil, 1 tbsp	0
Potato salad, 1 tbsp	28
Salad cream, 100g	16.7
Thousand island dressing, 1 tbsp	3.5
Thousand island dressing, light, 1 tbsp	3.5

FISH & FISH PRODUCTS	
Cod in batter, fried, 100g	7.5
Cod, grilled, poached or baked, 100g	0
Eel, 100g	0
Fish fingers, grilled, per finger, average	5.4
Herring, grilled, 100g	0
Lemon sole, 100g	0

FOOD	Carbs grams
FISH & FISH PRODUCTS CONTINUED	
Lumpfish, 100g	0
Mussels, 100g	0
Pilchards, canned in tomato sauce, 100g	0.7
Prawns, boiled, 100g	0
Salmon, 100g	0
Salmon, smoked, 100g	0
Sardines, canned in oil, drained, 100g	0
Sardines, fresh, 100g	0.5
Scampi, breaded and fried, 100g	28.9
Trout, rainbow, 100g	0
Tuna, canned, brine/water and drained, 100g	0
Tuna, canned in oil, drained, 100g	0

FRUIT	
Apples, average, flesh and skin, 100g	11.8
Apricots, 100g	36.5
Avocado, average, flesh only, 100g	1.9
Bananas, no skin, 100g	23.2
Figs, dried, 100g	52.9
Grapefruit, flesh only, 100	6.8
Grapes, seedless, 100g	15.4
Kiwi fruit, whole, 100g	10.6
Fruit salad, canned in syrup, drained, 100g	11.5
Fruit salad, fresh, 100g	13.7
Mangoes, flesh only, 100g	14.1
Melon, honeydew, flesh only, 100g	6.6
Oranges, flesh only, 100g	8.5
Peaches, whole, 100g	7.6
Peaches, canned in syrup, 100g	14
Pears, whole, 100g	9.1
Pineapple, canned in juice, 100g	12.2
Plums, whole, average, 100g	8.3
Prunes, 100g	34
Strawberries, 100g	6

FOOD	Carbs grams
MILK & YOGURTS	
Condensed milk, sweetened, 250ml	138.8
Evaporated milk, full fat, 250ml	21.3
Full fat milk, 250ml	12
Muller rice, low-fat, 200g	28
Semi-skimmed milk, 250ml	12.5
Skimmed milk, 250ml	12.5
Soya milk, 250ml	22.5
Yogurt, whole milk, plain, 200g	15.6
Yogurt, low-fat, fruit, 150g	26.8

MEAT & MEAT PRODUCTS	
Bacon, rashers, 2, 38g	0
Bacon, rashers, lean, 2, 32,	0
Beef, steak, grilled, 100g	0
Beef, mince, 100g	0
Beef burgers, frozen, fried, 100g	7
Beef, fillet steak, lean and trimmed, grilled, 100g	0
Black pudding, fried, 100g	15
Chicken breast, no skin, grilled, 100g	0
Chicken breast, with skin, grilled, 100g	1

FOOD	Carbs grams
MEAT & MEAT PRODUCTS CONTINUED	
Corned beef, canned, 100g	0
Ham, canned, 100g	0
Ham, slices, no added water, 1 slice, 25g	0.2
Lamb chop, lean grilled, 100g	0
Lamb chop, untrimmed, grilled, 100g	0
Lamb shank, lean, 100g	0
Pork crackling, 30g	0
Pork fillet, lean grilled, 100g	0
Pork loin chop, fat trimmed off, grilled, 100g	0
Pork loin, untrimmed, grilled, 100g	0
Pork pie, 180g	44.8
Salami, 100g	1.9
Sausages, beef, grilled, 100g	15.2
Sausages, pork, grilled, 100g	11.5
Sausages, pork extra lean, 100g	10.8
Steak and kidney pie, 100g	25.6
Turkey, oven cooked, lean, 100g	0
Turkey, breast, no skin, 100g	0
Veal, loin chop, grilled, 100g	4.4
Veal, schnitzel, 100g	10
Veal, shank, lean, 100g	0

NUTS	
Almonds, flesh only, 100g	6.9
Almonds, chocolate coated, 100g	66
Brazil, 100g	3.1
Cashew, 100g	27.9
Hazelnuts, 100g	6
Mixed nuts, 100g	7.6
Mixed nuts and raisins, 100g	31.5
Peanuts, roasted and salted, 100g	7.1
Pecan, 100g	5.8

FOOD	Carbs grams
PASTA	
Egg, cooked, 100g	25.5
Plain, all shapes, cooked, 100g	24.7
Ravioli, cheese and spinach, cooked, 100g	33.2
Spinach, cooked, 100g	27.2
Ravioli, cheese & spinach, cooked, 100g	19.6
Tomato and herb fettuccine, 100g	33.2
Tortollini, cheese and spinach, cooked, 100g	23.3
Wholemeal, cooked, 100g	23.2

PASTRY	
Filo, 1 sheet	7.5
Flaky, 100g	45.9
Puff, 100g	27
Shortcrust, 100g	54.2
Wholemeal, 100g	44.6

POTATO & POTATO PRODUCTS	
Baked potato, medium, 150g	47.6
Boiled, potatoes, 150g	26.7
Chips, homemade, fried in oil, 100g	30.1
Chips, oven baked, frozen, 100g	29.8
Mashed with skimmed milk, 100g	14
Roasted with skin, 100g	25.9

FOOD	Carbs grams
PUDDINGS & DESSERTS	
Apple pie, shop bought, 100g	56.7
Apple pie, low-fat, 100g	32
Apple strudel, 100g	41
Bread pudding, 100g	49.7
Cheesecake, frozen, 100g	33
Chocolate mousse, 100g	19.9
Chocolate sponge, 100g	54.4
Custard made with whole milk, 100g	16.6
Christmas pudding, 100g	49.5
Custard tart, 100g	32.4
Fruit crumble, 100g	34
Fruit pie, pastry top and bottom, 100g	34
Lemon meringue pie, 100g	45.9
Pecan pie, 100g	56
Rice pudding, canned, 100g	14
Soufflé, 100g	10.5
Tiramisu, 100g	0
Trifle, 100g	22.3

SAUCES	
SAUCES	
Bolognaise, 100g	3.7
Gravy, commercial, 100g	2.9
Hungarian goulash, 100g	6.6
Oyster, 1 tbsp	3.4
Pesto, 1 tbsp	9
Sweet & sour, 1 serving 115g	30.5

FOOD	Carbs grams
TOFU	
Fried, 100g	2
Burgers, 100g	0
Veggie burgers, 100g	0

VEGETABLES	
Aubergine, 100g	2.2
Beans, baked, canned in tomato sauce, 100g	13.3
Beans, red kidney, canned, drained, 100g	8.8
Beetroot, boiled, 100g	9.5
Brussels sprouts, 100g	4.1
Cabbage, raw, average, 100g	4.1
Carrots, old, boiled, 100g	4.9
Cauliflower, boiled, 100g	2.1
Courgette, raw, 100g	1.8
Cucumber, 100g	1.5
Lentils, red dried, 100g	56.3
Mushrooms, raw, 100g	0.4
Peas, frozen, 100g	11.3
Peppers, green, raw, 100g	2.6
Spinach, frozen, 100g	0.5
Sweet potato, 100g	21.5
Sweetcorn kernels, canned, 100g	26.6
Tofu, soya bean, 100g	0.7
Tomatoes, raw, 100g	3.1
Turnip, boiled, 100g	2
Watercress, 100g	0.4

YORKSHIRE PUDDING	
Small, 50g	12.4

FAST FOOD OUTLETS	Carbs grams
BURGER KING	
Angus steak burger, 1, 276g	59
Bacon Cheeseburger, 1, 141g	31
Bagel, egg, cheese, sausage, 1, 203g	50
Chicken club, 1, 242g	54
Chicken fries, 6 pieces, 85g	18
Chicken whopper, 1, 272g	48
Veggie burger, 1, 272g	47
KENTUCKY FRIED CHICKEN	
Blazing twister s/w, 1, 246g	56
Chicken fillet burger, 1, 213g	40.5
Chicken pot pie, 1 serving, 243g	70
Crispy twister s/w, 1, 252g	55
Kentucky nuggets, 6 nuggets	0
Medium fries, 100g	36
McDONALD'S	
Bagel, ham, egg, cheese, 1, 218g	58
Big breakfast, 266g	53
Big Mac, 1, 219g	47
Cheeseburger, 1, 119g	35
Chicken McNuggets, 10 nuggets,	26
Medium fries, 100g	47

FAST FOOD OUTLETS	Carbs grams
PIZZA HUT	
BBQ wings starter, per serving	6.7
Chicken and bacon salad, per serving	22.4
Lasagne, per serving	64
Muffin, mixed berry, 1	44.9
Pizza, farmhouse, medium pan, per serving	27.3
Pizza, Hawaiian, stuffed crust, per serving	30.6
Pizza, Margherita, medium pan, per serving	27.3

SUBWAY SANDWICHES	
6" Bourbon chicken, 1, 258g	54
6" Cheese steak, toasted, 1, 250g	47
6" Cheese and bacon ranch, 1, 296	47
6" Subway club, 1, 256g	47
6" Subway melt, 1, 254g	48
6" Tuna, 1, 250g	45

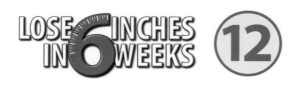

WATCH OUT
FOR
THE SABOTEURS

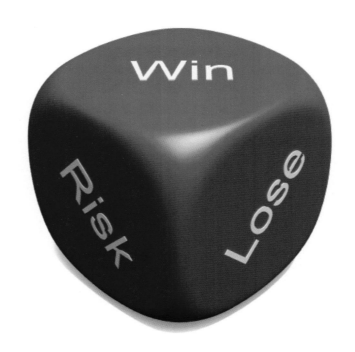

ALCOHOL

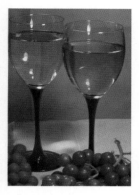

Fat does not always work alone; he sometimes has a friend, a pal, a partner in crime. When these two guys get together, they can inflict some serious damage. They are the ideal team to create havoc to your inch-loss plans. What's more, this accomplice has the potential to cause further harm the following day. The other member of this deadly duo is alcohol!

You have been invited to a meal around your friends house where you have just finished the pudding. The wine has been flowing all night and the conversation is still going strong. You've lost count of the number of times your wine glass has been topped up and you are feeling very relaxed. Then suddenly the cheese and biscuits appear. It's not that often that you enjoy cheese and biscuits at the end of a meal, so you decide to make a little more room in your tummy to treat yourself to some.

When you look at your wine glass, you discover it's nearly empty. How can you possible enjoy cheese and biscuits without a glass of wine? The only difference is that you don't have to make any room in your tummy for the wine.

Alcohol can be viewed as many things, from something to help you relax, to an essential part of any meal or social occasion. Interestingly, alcohol is not usually something seen as food but it is.

Alcohol is liquid food, except that unlike solid food,
it will not curb your hunger and it has a low nutritional value.

SENSIBLE DRINKING LEVELS

Alcohol is measured in units.
Current daily sensible drinking guidelines for adults are:
Females: 2-3 units or less   Males: 3-4 units or less
Refraining on one day should not mean excess on another

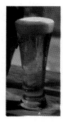

1 unit of alcohol is a
half pint of standard beer (3.5%vol)

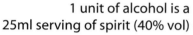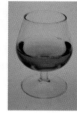

1 unit of alcohol is a
25ml serving of spirit (40% vol)

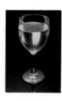

One small glass of wine
(125ml) contains 1.5 units of alcohol

WHAT'S IN YOUR DRINK?

The calories within alcoholic drinks come from two sources, which are alcohol and sugar. Most alcoholic drinks carry no calories from fat. However, cream liqueurs and some cocktails do contain fat, which is in the cream. The table below is just a general guideline to the content of popular alcoholic drinks and this can vary depending upon their volume of alcohol.

Description	Alcohol Content	Sugar Content	Total Calories
500ml can of low-alcohol beer	15.5g	11.5g	152
500ml can of sweet cider	26g	21.5g	262
Half bottle of red wine	36g	1g	256
Half bottle of dry white wine	34g	2g	245
Half bottle of sweet white wine	38g	22g	351
Small glass of red wine (125ml)	12g	.5g	86
Small glass of dry white wine (125ml)	11g	.75g	82
Small glass of sweet white wine (125ml)	13g	7g	117
Spirits (Double)	16g	Nil	143

ALCOHOL & EXERCISE

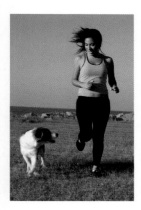

Unlike fat and carbohydrate, which are both used as energy inside your muscles, alcohol is not. Although you may think that you can exercise for 30 to 60 minutes and sweat out the calories from alcohol, unfortunately, alcohol cannot be used as energy by your muscles.

Dietitians in Sport & Exercise Nutrition
"Although alcohol has a high-energy content, it is not used for exercise, as it is broken down in the liver not the muscles. If your total energy intake is higher than your output, it will contribute indirectly to extra weight gain as fat deposits"

BINGE DRINKING
A heavy drinking session can increase calorie intake by up to an additional 2,000 calories. Regular binge drinking at the weekend will take its toll, as this type of lifestyle behaviour will show within a couple of years. This is especially true for teenagers who start drinking young.

ALCOHOL – THE DOUBLED EDGED SWORD
As previously discussed alcohol is liquid food and the more alcohol you drink, the fewer calories from food you should consume. However, the reality is that the more alcohol you drink the poorer choices you will probably make for meals and snacks.

If you have drunk excessively the night before this will probably impinge on your activity levels the next day. How quickly do you move around with a hangover?

In this way, alcohol can be seen as a doubled edged sword. It cuts because of the additional calories consumed at the time and again the next day through lower activity levels.

CONTROL ALCOHOL INTAKE

Next to fat, controlling your alcohol intake is one of the best ways to see really fast results in both the way you look and feel. If you do drink alcohol on a regular basis then look to follow these guidelines.

- Plan to have at least two nights that are alcohol free each week.
- Buy in some low-calorie drinks as an alternative to alcohol.
- Adopt the habit of drinking at least one pint of water after you have been drinking alcohol.
- Offer to be the driver on any social occasions and don't drink alcohol. This also takes off any peer pressure to drink.
- Realise that the size of your glass can make a difference and look to use a smaller glass as your guide to controlling units.

ALCOHOL	Women Points Lost	Men Points Lost
Up to 2 units/day	0	0
Up to 3 units/day	1	0
4 units/day	2	1
6 units/day	3	2
8 units/day	4	3
10 units/day	5	4
11 units/day		5

Plan to have at least two days a week that are alcohol free. You can have an additional two units on Fridays & Saturdays without losing any points.

Remember that every large glass of wine you drink you are consuming nearly 150 calories.

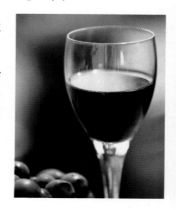

By good personal management of your units of alcohol you are controlling your calorie intake without counting calories. Again this is where your Score Card puts you in control of alcohol every day.

SLEEP

In the mid eighties I held the position of The Army Athletic Specialist at the Army School of Physical Training in Aldershot. This was and still is a place where students are enthusiastically encouraged to move from one class to the next very quickly.

One of the very good army women runners at the time approached me and asked if I would give her some help with her running programme. Maggie, who was Welsh, wanted one last chance to make the Welsh Womens' Cross Country Team.

I knew Maggie very well. She was a really tough individual and competitor who would willingly give 100 percent in training. I also was aware that Maggie liked to go clubbing every weekend. I said that I would be delighted to help her...under one condition. She asked me what that was. I said that she would need to give up clubbing at the weekends. Maggie asked me why.

I explained that from what I had seen of her training, there were only a few recommendations that I felt would make a difference to the technical content of her training. However, giving one hundred percent during training on Sundays, Mondays and Tuesdays may sound great. Except, she was giving 100 percent of the energy she had available on those days. Because of her clubbing this was not 100 percent of her potential. It was taking Maggie until Wednesday before she could tap into her true potential. She was under-performing in training three days every week because of her late nights at the weekend.

Maggie said that she had never thought about it in this way before and she agreed and kept her part of the bargain. Maggie successfully made the Womens' Welsh Cross Country Team that year. Incidentally, just before I moved on from the Army School of Physical Training I was told about a young lance corporal coming through, who some said, would soon challenge Maggie. I thought to myself that she will probably not be good enough and certainly not tough enough. Her name was lance corporal Kelly Holmes!

What do I know about running anyway?

LIFESTYLE

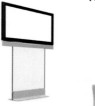

The amount of sleep you need is specific to you as an individual with the average being around eight hours every 24 hours.

It is a fact that our lifestyles have changed dramatically over the last 30 years and this has impinged on the amount of sleep we get. We now sit down and watch nearly twice as much TV as we did 30 years ago. We now stay up much later, gazing into an ever increasing size of box. Then include the amount of time we spend sitting down surfing the net in the evening and there are just so many distractions to keep you away from getting a good night's sleep through the week.

Also, take into consideration that we have the opportunity to play for much longer at the weekends. It is very easy to find a pub open to the wee hours in the mornings in most towns. Pill popping to keep bodies active and squeeze that bit more out of the weekend is common place, especially for the clubbing culture. Yet there is a toll to be paid for this type of lifestyle. The Monday morning feeling is not helped by late nights on Friday or Saturday. Then it is back to relaxing in front of the box or surfing the web again. It can become a vicious circle.

Lack of sleep affects your body in a number of ways. The most obvious sign is a general feeling of tiredness during the day. This is a precursor to a breakdown in willpower, leading to poor decision making regarding meals and snacks. In addition, you gain less benefit out of any exercise workout, exercise class or gym session through lower energy levels. If you do exercise when you are feeling really tired, then you are more susceptible to injury or illness.

As the example of Maggie on the previous page shows, you can be working harder for less benefit. Even if you're eating sensibly and being active you must ensure you get enough sleep for you to achieve your true potential.

If you are a parent with the responsibility of having young children, can you imagine letting them stay up as long as they wanted to watch TV? Then expect them to wake bright eyed and full of enthusiasm for the day ahead ready to achieve their potential?

PROFESSOR JIM HORNE
"Correct sleep is a necessity which is hazardous to ignore."

Sleep is something that most of us take for granted. To look and feel good about yourself, and, achieve your true potential, then getting enough sleep should become one of your priorities.

TAKE RESPONSIBILITY
No one except you can tell you what time to go to bed. In this way you need to take responsibility for deciding on a time and make sure that you stick to it.

THE TV
Decide what programmes you really want to watch, ideally plan this for the whole week. Then switch the TV off once you have seen your programmes.

FALLING ASLEEP EARLY EVENING
This can easily become a habit, especially at the end of a long tiring day. You may feel physically exhausted but in reality you could be emotionally tired. This habit can lead to going to bed that bit later in the evening and then waking up in the morning feeling tired.

Look to take a shower and get changed into different clothes. Try to have a cup of tea or coffee to stimulate you. Definitely avoid the situation of sitting down watching a programme on the TV in a comfortable chair as soon as you get home.

PHYSICAL ACTIVITY
If you intend to step up your present physical activity levels, then you should also look at getting to bed a little earlier on those days.

THE BENEFITS OF ENOUGH SLEEP

- You rejuvenate your body and mind

- You wake up refreshed ready for the challenges of a new day

- You can focus on the task in hand much easier

- You are able to make better decisions and choices

- You communicate better, especially with those closest to you

- Your physical potential is improved and you see results sooner

- You recover from any workout much faster

- Your ego is recharged and your self esteem boosted

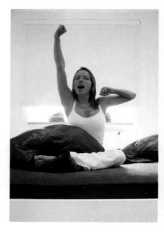

Only you will know if you are currently getting enough sleep. The table below gives you the opportunity to record your sleep for one week.

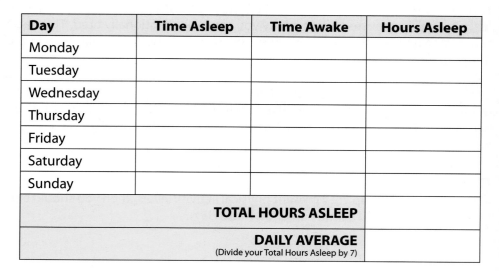

Day	Time Asleep	Time Awake	Hours Asleep
Monday			
Tuesday			
Wednesday			
Thursday			
Friday			
Saturday			
Sunday			
		TOTAL HOURS ASLEEP	
		DAILY AVERAGE (Divide your Total Hours Asleep by 7)	

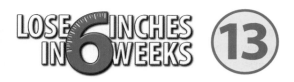

13

THE MAINTENANCE PLAN

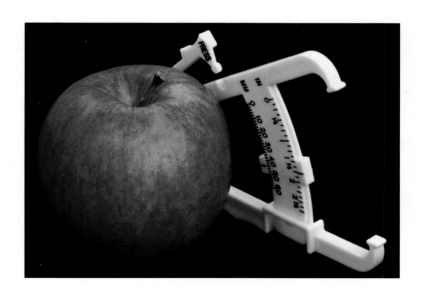

YOUR FIRST STEP

The first step is for you to lose at least 6 inches of fat in the next 6 weeks. At the end of this initial 6 week period you have choices. You can continue to use this score card to lose more inches or you can use your score card as part of your maintenance plan. The average inch loss with the IntaShape Plan for the first 6 weeks is shown below.

HEIGHT	AVERAGE WEEKLY SCORE TO LOSE 6 INCHES IN 6 WEEKS
Taller than 184cm Taller than 6ft	An average of at least 48 points
171cm -184cm 5ft 7in to 6ft	An average of at least 50 points
164cm – 171cm 5ft 4in to 5ft 7in	An average of at least 52 points
155cm – 164cm 5ft 1in to 5ft 4in	An average of at least 54 points
Smaller than 155cm Smaller than 5ft 1in	An average of at least 56 points

To continue to lose inches all you need to do is score yourself the same weekly average for another 6 weeks. Holidays, the festive season are all times when we tend to add on a few extra inches. All you need to do is use this score card and hit the same weekly average to start dropping inches once again.

MAINTENANCE PLAN

Once you have decided that you have lost enough inches, then you can use the score card again to help you keep those inches off through the maintenance plan. To keep the inches off all you need to do is to drop your average weekly score by around 6 points a week as follows:

THE INTASHAPE MAINTENANCE PLAN

HEIGHT	AVERAGE WEEKLY SCORE TO LOSE 6 INCHES IN 6 WEEKS
Taller than 184cm Taller than 6ft	An average of at least 42 points
171cm -184cm 5ft 7in to 6ft	An average of at least 44 points
164cm – 171cm 5ft 4in to 5ft 7in	An average of at least 46 points
155cm – 164cm 5ft 1in to 5ft 4in	An average of at least 48 points
Smaller than 155cm Smaller than 5ft 1in	An average of at least 50 points

For more information visit our website…
www.intashape.com

6 WEEK SCORE CARD

THE PLAN FOR FOOD & DRINKS

Low Fat
Breakfast

Morning
Snack

Low Fat
Lunch

Afternoon
Snack

Low Fat
Evening Meal

Evening Snack
(Optional)

2-3 Units

FOOD & DRINKS SECTION

	Day 1	Day 2	Day 3	Day 4	Day 5	Day 6	Day 7	FOOD & DRINK SCORE
Week 1	+	+	+	+	+	+	=	
Week 2	+	+	+	+	+	+	=	
Week 3	+	+	+	+	+	+	=	
Week 4	+	+	+	+	+	+	=	
Week 5	+	+	+	+	+	+	=	
Week 6	+	+	+	+	+	+	=	

ACTIVITY SECTION

	Day 1	Day 2	Day 3	Day 4	Day 5	Day 6	Day 7	ACTIVITY SCORE	COMBINED SCORE
Week 1	+	+	+	+	+	+	=		
Week 2	+	+	+	+	+	+	=		
Week 3	+	+	+	+	+	+	=		
Week 4	+	+	+	+	+	+	=		
Week 5	+	+	+	+	+	+	=		
Week 6	+	+	+	+	+	+	=		